Avian Malaria

in the

Asian Tropical Subregion

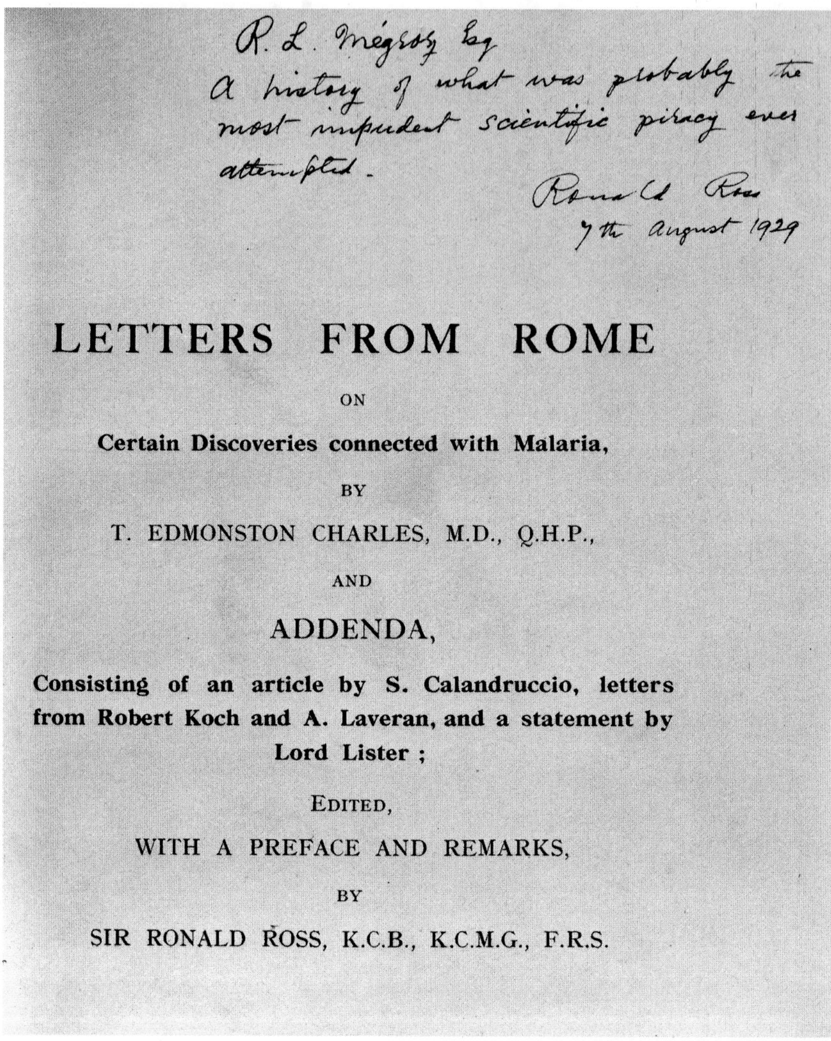

R. L. Mégroz Esq
A history of what was probably the most impudent scientific piracy ever attempted.
Ronald Ross
7th August 1929

LETTERS FROM ROME

ON

Certain Discoveries connected with Malaria,

BY

T. EDMONSTON CHARLES, M.D., Q.H.P.,

AND

ADDENDA,

Consisting of an article by S. Calandruccio, letters from Robert Koch and A. Laveran, and a statement by Lord Lister ;

EDITED,

WITH A PREFACE AND REMARKS,

BY

SIR RONALD ROSS, K.C.B., K.C.M.G., F.R.S.

Inscribed title page to Sir Ronald Ross's presentation copy to his biographer, R. L. Mégroz, of the 1929 edition of his *Letters from Rome…* (see Preface, p. xii).

Avian Malaria

in the

Asian Tropical Subregion

With 138 photomicrographs

Marshall Laird MSc (Hons), PhD, DSc, FAAAS

Springer

Marshall Laird, MSc (Hons), PhD, DSc, FAAAS
"Awawhare"
Pahi Road
RD 1
Paparoa 1240
New Zealand

Library of Congress Cataloging-in-Publication Data

Laird, Marshall.
Avian malaria in the Asian tropical subregion / Marshall Laird.
p. cm.
Includes bibliographical references (p.).
ISBN 9813083190
1. Avian malaria--Asia. 2. Plasmodium--Asia. 3. Avian malaria--Tropics.
4. Plasmodium--Tropics. I. Title.
SF995.6.M3L35 1997
636.5'08969362--dc21 97-11057
CIP

ISBN 981-3083-19-0

Front cover illustration: A schizont of *Plasmodium nucleophilum*, tightly pressed against the nucleus of a parasitized erythrocyte of a weaverbird from Thailand (see Figure 7.27).

Typesetting: Expo Holdings Sdn Bhd
Printed in Singapore
SPIN 10576370 5 4 3 2 1

To the late Prof. P. C. C. Garnham, CMG, FRS,

without whose gentle reminders of recent years
the completion of this book would have been rather less likely.

Preface

For millennia human malaria was a leading cause of fever and death. It remains so, despite the World Health Organization's Malaria Eradication Programme from the late 1950s to the early 1970s, and its promise of Health for All by the Year 2000.

Four species of the protozoan genus *Plasmodium* collectively account for humankind's share of the disease most widely known as malaria (Italian for "bad air", derived from marshland miasmata). The malady's French name, *paludisme*, specifically relates it to the marshes themselves, rather than their supposedly noxious effluvia. In English, malaria was included in the meaning of "ague", which from the fourteenth century if not earlier signified "an acute or violent fever".

But long before the emergence of these modern languages, the Greeks of the fourth century BC had already recognized the chief varieties of malaria from their clinical symptoms (Jones 1907); while the link between the disease, standing water and mosquitoes emerging from it to bite humans had been suspected in ancient times. Thus in an Indian Veda (to introduce the Asian Tropical Subregion to these general introductory remarks) there was "a recognizable description of malaria and the suggestion that mosquitoes might carry diseases, possibly that which causes chills and fever" (Russell 1955). Other such perceptive speculation persisted over the ensuing centuries.

The problem's eventual elucidation necessarily had to await the scientific revolution and in particular, the development of high-power microscopy. So equipped, a French army medical officer, Major Alfonse Laveran (1880), became the first to recognize one of the human malaria parasites. On 6 November 1880 he saw the crescentic gametocytes of what is now known as *Plasmodium falciparum* in blood freshly drawn from a malarious soldier in Algeria. Next day he witnessed the exflagellation of (male) microgametocytes that had become freed from host erythrocytes in the victim's standing blood — in the normal course of events this process and the subsequent fertilization of (female) macrogametocytes must await the ingestion of infected blood by a suitable anopheline mosquito. This, though, was not to be demonstrated for almost two decades.

Four years afterwards, and altogether unaware of Laveran's discovery, Danilewsky (1884) observed such exflagellation of what he called *Polymitus* (actually a *Plasmodium*, this generic name not being proposed, by Marchiafava and Celli, until the following year) from wild birds at Kharkov, Ukraine.

Danilewsky thereby became, as Garnham (1966) declared, "the first to demonstrate the wide distribution of these parasites in the animal kingdom".

Garnham's classical volume minutely details subsequent developments in this fascinating history, in which a number of Italian scientists were brilliantly involved. The name *Plasmodium* was first applied by Marchiafava and Celli (1885) to the causal agent of Malignant Tertian (MT) malaria, which did not receive its specific identity as *falciparum* until bestowed by Welch (1897). Grassi and Feletti (1890) gave the Benign Tertian (BT) parasite its specific name of *vivax*, the intraerythrocytic stages of this species having already been differentiated from those of Quartan malaria by Golgi (1885). The latter species duly became *malariae* thanks to Grassi and Feletti (1892). As reference to Garnham (1966) will show, there had been much nomenclatural confusion over the three chief human malaria parasites up to that point. A fourth and relatively rare although widely distributed species, *P. ovale*, was added by Stephens (1922); and a move by Garnham (1953) and Bray (1958) to break up the by-then quite large genus *Plasmodium* into separate genera proved "generally unwelcome".

The latter words are those of Garnham (1966), who went on to state that: "The case of subgeneric names has, however, much in its favour and was the course of action recommended by Corradetti, Garnham and Laird (1963) for the avian parasites", thereby preserving the generic name *Plasmodium* "available for general use". Bray (1963) had already followed suit by introducing the subgenera *Plasmodium* and *Laverania* for the mammalian malaria parasites, while Garnham (1964) had split off the species from subprimates as subgenus *Vinckeia*.

To accord them their full scientific names, the human malaria parasites are thus currently classified as:

- *Plasmodium (Plasmodium) vivax* (Grassi and Feletti 1890)
- *Plasmodium (Plasmodium) malariae* (Grassi and Feletti 1892)
- *Plasmodium (Plasmodium) ovale* Stephens 1922
- *Plasmodium (Laverania) falciparum* (Welch 1897).

For any unfamiliar with the International Code of Zoological Nomenclature, when the original describers' names and the relevant date of publication appear within parentheses, this signifies that the generic name originally used has since been emended. Thus in the first instance above, *P. vivax* was initially placed with the genus *Haemamoeba*, proposed by Grassi and Feletti for the malaria parasites of both humans and birds. It was later agreed that the generic name *Plasmodium* applied by Marchiafava and Celli (1885) to what is now known as *Plasmodium falciparum* (the most dangerous of the human malaria parasites) should serve for all agents of malaria, whether human or not; *Haemamoeba* being reserved as a subgeneric name for certain of the species parasitizing birds (see p. 23).

But to continue, although Danilewsky (1884; 1889) was the first to discover true malaria parasites in birds, the first valid description was that of "*Haemamoeba relicta*", now *Plasmodium (Haemamoeba) relictum* (Grassi and Feletti 1891). Their type host was the Spanish Sparrow in Catania, Sicily (see p. 27). On present evidence this is the world's most widely distributed malaria parasite, with a greater host range than any other. It "is a virulent parasite which causes an unknown amount of damage to the bird life of the world".

That quotation is from Garnham (1966), who described a 1905 incident illustrating how the importation of non-immune birds into a malarious population suffering little mortality can strike down the newcomers. In this instance, 100 partridges were imported into France in 1905 to augment the game on a proprietor's shoot. They rapidly sickened with newly acquired infections of a strain of *P. relictum* new to them, and all were soon dead. Garnham stated that at the peak of serious infections the sufferers looked ill, with ruffled plumage ... and displayed a markedly hypertrophied liver and spleen. Some 80 years earlier, Danilewsky (1889–91) had already recognized these and other consequences of *Plasmodium* infection in his pioneer investigations of bird malaria; which now ceased, the taxonomic placement of *Plasmodium relictum* by Grassi and Feletti already referred to being followed by a few years in which the human malaria parasites were at the centre of attention.

Ronald Ross, a surgeon in the Indian Medical Service (IMS) now entered the malariological arena. While Garrison-Surgeon at Bangalore in the spring of 1884, he had begun to take an interest in the control of pest culicine mosquitoes utilizing various kinds of artificial containers as larval habitats, but according to his biographer (Mégroz 1931) he was then giving serious attention to switching from medicine to literature as a profession — a man of wide interests, he was particularly attracted to verse in that period. However, on leave in London in 1894–95, he won the triennial Parkes Memorial Prize for the latter year "for the best essay on malaria", much of this being "devoted to demolishing ... the old theory that malaria was a kind of exhalation from damp areas such as marshes, and it was therefore caught by breathing" (Mégroz 1931).

During this home leave, Patrick Manson (the discoverer in 1877 of the mosquito phase of the filarial worm *Wuchereria bancrofti*) demonstrated malaria parasites to Ross in the blood of a London hospital patient. Ross also learnt of the informed conjectures of King (1883) and Laveran (1884) that mosquitoes might well prove to transmit *Plasmodium*, too. Now motivated to investigate this question himself, he returned to India later in 1895 and was soon examining exflagellating microgametocytes in malarious human blood. No trained zoologist, though, in his continuing correspondence with Manson he was still referring to the freed gametes as "flagella" despite Golgi's (1889) revelation of their true nature in his investigations at Pavia.

Without knowledge of the systematics of Culicidae, he then proceeded to rear from the larval stage (or "grub" as he styled it) brindled, grey and spotted-winged mosquitoes. After feeding from malaria patients, these were dissected and searched for *Plasmodium* — but to no avail. This is understandable in retrospect, for until the spring of 1897 he had only encountered a single spotted-winged mosquito. Moreover, in mitigation of his imprecision concerning mosquito identities, although the genera *Culex* and *Anopheles* were first described in 1758 and 1818, respectively, Russell (1955) explained that, until 1886 in the former case and 1896 in the latter, good English descriptions of these were unavailable. Besides, by no means every species of *Anopheles* can transmit human malaria, and some non-anophelines have variously spotted wings.

However, the adult Culicidae that laboratory assistant Mahomet Bux brought to Ross at Secunderabad on 16 August 1897 were indeed anophelines. About a dozen of them had been reared from larvae, and were now "fed on a malarious patient and put each in a test-tube" (Mégroz 1931). Through misadventure only three (one dead and decayed) remained by the morning of 20 August. That afternoon Ross discovered rounded, pigmented bodies "of about 12 microns in diameter" on the outer stomach wall of one of the survivors. Next day he was able to demonstrate growth of such bodies, the largest of them being some 20 μm in diameter, on dissecting the second and last-surviving anopheline. In the words of Garnham (1966), "This experiment constituted the first demonstration of the early stages in the development of *P. falciparum* in the mosquito." Its results were briefly published before the end of the year (Ross 1897). While the discovery "made it practically certain that mosquitoes, very likely *Anopheles*, transmit human malaria" (Russell 1955), and Ross was already beginning to seek final proof of this, he was suddenly transferred to quite another project, ending up in Calcutta in February 1898. Although authorized to resume malariological investigations there, he found it impracticable to work with human volunteers for reasons apparently associated with rioting arising from the use of "Mr. Haffkine's anti-plague inoculation" according to Russell (1955).

A year or more earlier Ross had received Patrick Manson's letter of 12 October 1896, declaring as cited by Manson-Bahr and Alcock (1927, p. 149) that were he himself tropically based he would pursue what we now know as plasmodial microgametocyte exflagellation in avian rather than human parasites — his reasons ranged from likely better access to bird malaria than to *P. falciparum*, to avoidance of possible homicide accusations in the event of his experiments terminating fatally with respect to the vertebrate host! Ross now followed this advice, having found that culicines (called "grey mosquitoes" by him, and latterly identified as expatriate American *Culex quinquefasciatus*) and peridomestic passerines both abounded in Calcutta. Using what Garnham (1966) and others afterwards believed to be *Plasmodium relictum* as his avian malaria subject, Ross (1898) now proceeded to expose naturally parasitized larks and sparrows (of an Asian race of *Passer domesticus*) to the hoped-for vector — doubtless spurred on by Manson's nationalism that led him to urge the India Office on 5 July 1897 that "in tropical diseases, Frenchmen, Italians, Germans, Americans, and even Japanese, are shooting ahead of us" (Manson-Bahr and Alcock 1927, p. 156).

Ross's first infection attempt took place on 11/12 March 1898. His subsequent examinations of the mosquitoes that fed, revealed a single example with "pigmented cells" (= oocysts) on the outer stomach wall. The possible donor was tracked back to three of the larks and a sparrow.

On the night of 17/18 March three larks were exposed to numerous grey mosquitoes, nine of which proved engorged on 20 March. Five of these exhibited oocysts on dissection. Feeling that his findings were almost conclusive, from 18 March to 21 May he fed his grey mosquitoes on four groups of birds. Group (a) involved larks, sparrows and a crow with *Plasmodium*; group (b) crows, pigeons and other birds with only halteridium (= *Haemoproteus*); group (c) a lark and a sparrow with immature *Plasmodium* only; and group (d) with a single healthy sparrow. He declared that "Only the insects fed on group (a) have contained pigmented cells" (i.e. today's oocysts).

This was proof positive of the culicine mosquito acquisition of avian malaria. Ross sent an advance copy of his paper to Manson, who read it on 24 July at the Edinburgh Meeting of the British Medical Association; by which time telegraphic communications from Ross had shown that the growing oocysts project into the host's body cavity, then burst to set free "germinal vermicules" (= sporozoites) which make their way to the salivary glands from which a duct leads into the proboscis. In Manson's (1898) paper on behalf of Ross, published on 20 August, Manson further stated that:

> *The climax of the discovery was now within his grasp and he elucidated it thus: He allowed mosquitoes to feed on birds infected with proteosoma; after a few days he fed the mosquitoes on birds whose blood was void of any parasite infection. He found in due course that the parasite-bearing mosquito had infected the healthy birds and that their blood was charged with proteosoma ... Thus the analogy between bird and human infection has only to be proved to establish that the mosquito is a carrier of malaria and an infector of man.*

For the first time the natural mode of transmission of malaria parasites had thus been demonstrated (Russell 1955; Garnham 1966).

Unhappily, despite the implications of this breakthrough, the IMS again interrupted the research by ordering Ross away from Calcutta on a kala-azar assignment. Returning to England in frustration he resigned from the IMS in June 1899 — and the great malaria controversy began. For the Italian scientists had continued their independent work "on the mosquito hypothesis all through these years" (Garnham 1966), and on 1 November 1898 Bignami, as the former author states, succeeded "in infecting a volunteer with *P. falciparum* by the bite of mosquitoes collected at Maccarese, a malarious locality near Rome". Giovanni Battista Grassi, a medically qualified zoologist who was then Prof. of Comparative Anatomy at the University of Rome, had (with Feletti) described *Plasmodium vivax* in 1890 and *P. malariae* in 1892, as already shown. It was his technician who had been regularly supplying Bignami and his colleague Bastianelli with the (culicine) mosquitoes they had used since 1894 in unproductive feeding experiments until he came back from Maccarese with adult females of *Anopheles claviger* at the end of October 1898.

In short order oocysts were now detected on *A. claviger* mid-gut walls, the cycle of development of both *P. falciparum* and *P. vivax* in mosquito vectors was elucidated, and the sporogony of *P. malariae* was described; the whole being published in what Garnham (1966) calls "Grassi's classic monograph" in 1900. Russell (1955) sums up the whole matter in declaring that while "to Ross is due, for all time, the credit of being first to place a scientific finger on mosquitoes as the agents that spread malaria from man to man ... To Italian workers must go great praise for applying Ross's avian discoveries so quickly to human malaria". Garnham (1966) unreservedly credits Ross with the discovery of "the natural mode of transmission of malaria parasites" in birds, only to be frustrated with respect to full demonstration of the human/anopheline cycle until "after the Italians had already completed the work in beautiful detail".

An angry Ross had now begun to accuse Grassi of pirating his discoveries. Accumulating testimonials from correspondents in Italy he had these privately printed in Liverpool in 1900 for circulation among friends as *Letters from Rome on the New Discoveries in Malaria*. This compilation's contents (not publicly issued for almost three decades) include allegations that Grassi was a rogue and a robber in scientific domains, and even that he and Italian collaborators not only ignored important details of Ross's published work but also invented their first infection experiments in Rome. Yet Russell (1955) insists that "Grassi and Celli, for example ... learned promptly of and gave full weight to Ross's proof of the transmission of avian malaria". However, the *Letters* had presumably influenced the Committee that awarded the Nobel Prize in Medicine for 1902 to Ross alone, rather than to him and Grassi as many had expected.

Clearly a brilliant and tenacious man, Ross also had remarkable mathematical talents. There were novels and books of verse to his credit too, and his useful handbook on mosquito control appeared in 1902. But his capacity for sustained and unreasonable anger shows in his bibliography by Mégroz (1931), the pre-publication text of which was authorized by him and in which Grassi's post-1898 papers on the mosquito theory are branded as consisting "mostly of guesswork (nearly all wrong) and prevarication". This hardly accords with the Royal Society of London's award to Grassi of the Darwin Medal in 1910, for zoological, including ichthyological, achievement! Grassi died in 1925, and pursuing him beyond the grave, Ross wrote the following presentation inscription to Mégroz on the title page of what became this author's own copy[1] of the first (1929) public issue of the *Letters*. Signed and dated 7th August 1929 it reads (see frontispiece): "A history of what was probably the most impudent scientific piracy ever attempted." It seems appropriate in view of the fast-approaching Centennial of these events to detail these matters here in the interest of objectivity in the relevant celebrations. It clearly did not pay to get on the wrong side of Ross, and there is a revealing admission by Mégroz (1931, p. 90) that "Ross, indeed, had to make himself a nuisance in Liverpool and London, *as he had formerly in India* [italics added by author], in his efforts to drive people into fruitful action". In a Service where orders were expected to be obeyed his IMS superiors may well have jumped at the chance of relieving themselves of a nuisance in despatching Ross on those field assignments that a more diplomatic man might have escaped; thereby avoiding being pipped at the post by Grassi and his co-workers in the race to prove the anopheline transmission of human malaria! The *avian* malaria breakthrough was nonetheless Ross's — Sir Ronald, following his 1911 honour of Knight Commander of the Bath.

MacCallum (1897) had become the first to unlock the secret of the exflagellation process, via a haematozoan relative of *Plasmodium*, a *Haemoproteus* from an Ontarian crow. His studies revealed that the "flagella" flung off by exflagellating microgametocytes fertilized macrogametocytes, leading to the "vermicule" (nowadays ookinete) stage, properly found in the vector's gut. But it was in cooling fresh blood preparations that MacCallum's ookinetes thrust their pointed end through the cell membrane of erythrocytes, as they were later shown to penetrate the (hippoboscid fly) vector's stomach wall.

This American student repeated his Canadian observation with *Plasmodium falciparum* ookinetes in blood slides from patients when he returned to complete his medical qualification in Baltimore. It was not long afterwards that Garnham, Bird and Baker (1962) confirmed matters by electron microscopy. MacCallum and his student friend Opie (1898) together initiated surveys of plasmodia in wild birds from various parts of the world (see Hewitt 1940, Table 1). The table, comprehensive up to that date, totals only 20 such surveys, and a total of 6916 birds with 5.8% positive for *Plasmodium*. The highest percentage of positives for an individual survey was that of Huff (1939) who

[1] Purchased following the early 1960s sale of the Mégroz library, and lately presented to The Library of the Wellcome Institute for the History of Medicine, 183 Euston Road, London, UK.

found *Plasmodium* in 18.2% of 324 birds of 32 species from various parts of the USA, and the lowest, that of Ogawa (1912) whose figure was 1% positives among 1478 birds of 54 species from Japan.

Of course such incidences are likely to show considerable variation, reflecting such factors as low host susceptibility, lack of immunity, presence and prevalence of suitable mosquito vectors, seasonal factors, etc. This is substantiated by more recent data reviewed by Garnham (1966), and an updated global host-parasite catalogue of avian malaria parasites and other haematozoa too, prepared by Bennett, Whiteway and Woodworth-Lynas (1982).

Although by the final years of the past century the intraerythrocytic and mosquito cycles of *Plasmodium* were no longer a mystery, it remained unknown where the parasites developed between the inoculation of sporozoites via the salivary ducts of mosquitoes into vertebrates, and the appearance after some delay of intraerythrocytic trophozoites in the circulation. Grassi (1900) hypothesized that during this incubation period there must be a third cycle of development within the parasitized vertebrate. For years now, avian malaria was central to the search for such a cycle, tissue stages of the exoerythrocytic phase being reported by several investigators before their true significance was realized by Raffaele (1934) in his studies of *Plasmodium elongatum*. Through and after World War II these investigations proceeded, with the exoerythrocytic cycle for malaria parasites of monkeys and then humans being revealed in liver parenchyma cells by Shortt and Garnham (1948) and Shortt *et al.* (1951). Once more Garnham (1966) should be referred to for a full account of these advances; and also of the leading role of bird malaria parasites, notably *P. relictum*, in the development of malaricidal drugs, concerning the earlier stages of which Hewitt (1940) remains a useful reference.

In recent years, though, the volume of such research has greatly diminished, and as reference to "Biological Abstracts" will show, investigations of avian plasmodia have fallen away markedly. Changing research priorities and fashions in science are at the same time highlighting the urgent need for biodiversity-related studies of the malaria parasites of birds. Although the potential of these for causing morbidity and sometimes severe mortality in their avian hosts had already been recognized by Danilewsky in the 1880s, who was the first to realize that such severity could be directly proportional to parasitaemia, the actual wiping out of a population has seldom been reported. And when it has, it has usually been due to the deliberate importation of birds into an area having a malaria parasite to which the local avifauna had acquired resistance but they had not. Examples are those of the Hungarian partridges already referred to as having speedily died after being brought to France (see Laveran and Lucet 1905) and the penguins from mosquito-free areas that have quickly succumbed when taken to distant zoos where avian plasmodia and suitable vectors were awaiting them (the first such instance was reported from the Gardens of the Zoological Society of London (Scott 1927) and others have followed). In these and similar instances the pathogen was usually confirmed as *P. relictum*.

Similar consequences involving a simuliid-transmitted relative of the plasmodia, *Leucocytozoon simondi*, were recorded in subarctic Quebec in the spring of 1959, when domestic Pilgrim Geese that the Canada Department of Agriculture was attempting to establish as year-round food for Inuit (Eskimos) were wiped out through infection by blackflies soon after the arrival from far south of large numbers of native ducks and geese in which migratory stress had maximized the number of gametocytes in their blood (Laird and Bennett 1970).

Also of much relevance is the fact that in Hawaii (altogether mosquito-free until 1826) Laysan Finches removed from their still mosquito-free remote outlier to the main islands where a subspecies of *P. relictum* has long been established, rapidly succumbed with massive parasitaemias when exposed to infection (Warner 1968; Laird and van Riper 1981). Nevertheless, on the large island of Hawaii itself, where avian malaria apparently did not reach epizootic proportions until about 1920, matters are otherwise. Although there has definitely been a negative impact on the population dynamics of the native forest birds, several of their species have now developed immunogenic and behavioural responses reducing the parasite's impact on their populations (van Riper *et al.* 1986). Complete recovery from astonishingly heavy infestations such as those illustrated by Laird and van Riper (1981) have also been noted.

Elsewhere for particularly the past two decades there has certainly been increasing awareness of the inexorably increasing pressures upon the global environment. This has centred upon human population growth and relevant pollution hazards, forest destruction (especially tropical) and the rest. But the significance in all this of avian malariology has been lost sight of. Work of undoubted value is now vigorously progressing in many of the more politically stable countries to save threatened ecosystems and particular groups of organisms — notably birds. But those devoting themselves to the latter have concentrated on threats (e.g. predator attack and habitat depletion) that are more obvious and newsworthy than *Plasmodium*.

Without a new wave of interest in the avian malaria parasites, for further investigations of which the Asian Tropical Subregion is uniquely suited by its location between the former Soviet Union's central Asian sector and Australasia, coupled with MAPS (p. 1) avian migration data (McClure 1974), many more at-risk birds may very soon be lost. For although presently possessing adequate biosystematic understanding of these parasites, we remain ignorant of their potential for finishing off those many avian species among the 1132 considered that are now known to harbour a diversity of haematozoa and to be already approaching the brink of extinction through habitat depletion, predation, etc., since the survey hereunder was conducted. And in particular, we still lack knowledge of all but a handful of the mosquito vectors involved. There is a real challenge here, especially for investigators based in the Subregion, to employ the data now presented to establish the pathological significance and relationships with migratory birds of a large percentage of the world's validated avian malaria parasites.

Acknowledgements

Sincere thanks are due to Dr. H. Elliott McClure and his former Migratory Animal Pathological Survey team for their provision of the huge collection of avian blood samples, the true malaria parasites of which are now belatedly reported upon. The field work was supported by the United States Army Research and Development Group (Far East) and the Walter Reed Army Institute of Research, Washington, DC, USA. A microscope lent by the former group enabled my initial (spare time) examination of many of the slides in Geneva. A former WHO colleague, the late Emeritus Prof. Leonard J. Bruce-Chwatt, CMG, OBE, had a major role in the designation of the WHO International Reference Centre for Avian Malaria Parasites at The Memorial University of Newfoundland in 1968, successive Presidents of which from 1968 to the mid-1990s supported the undertaking which duly evolved into the International Reference Centre for Avian Haematozoa headed by Prof. Gordon F. Bennett. Necessary equipment and research funding for my own relevant investigations were furnished by the National Research Council of Canada. Since my retirement to New Zealand, facilities have been generously provided by the School of Biological Sciences, University of Auckland; not least in arranging for the wordprocessing of the final draft onto hard disc by Miss Laurel Walker, for whose assistance (and forbearance!) I am most grateful.

Marshall Laird
May 1997

Summary

Eleven known species of *Plasmodium* and *P. (Novyella) corradettii* n.sp. are reported (and five others are queried) from 55 289 birds of 1132 species sampled from the Asian Tropical Subregion and bordering lands. The 538 individuals found positive for avian malaria represent 180 host species (15.9% of the total). They comprise 2.04% of the 26 385 examples of their hosts sampled and 0.97% of the overall collection. In 257 (47.8%) of the parasitized birds, plasmodial identification was impracticable below the generic level. Because of multiple infections, the remaining 281 positives were swollen to 364 species-determinations. These are of the following taxa, the number of infections for each being given in square brackets:

> *Plasmodium (Haemamoeba) relictum* **sensu lato** [41]; ssp. *relictum* [10]; ssp. *capistranoae* [2]; *P. (H.) cathemerium* [1 possible]; *P. (H.) matutinum* [44]; *P. (H.) giovannolai* [2 possibles]; *P. (Giovannolaia) fallax* [9]; *P. (G.) circumflexum* [6]; *P. (G.) polare* [27]; *P. (G.) lophurae* [1]; *P. (G.) dissanaikei* [31]; *P. (Novyella) vaughani* [75]; *P. (N.) rouxi* [75]; *P. (N.) nucleophilum* [32]; *P. (N.) corradettii* n.sp. [5]; *P. (Huffia) elongatum* [3].

An additional suspected finding is discarded as unlikely, *P. (H.) subpraecox* [1]. A wild (or feral?) Red Junglefowl from Palawan, Philippines, proved doubly parasitized by what on grounds of host-occurrence might well have been identified as *P. (H.) gallinaceum* and *P. (N.) juxtanucleare* (both already known from Domestic Fowl of the Asian Tropical Subregion). However, for both morphological and ecological reasons its parasites are determined as *P. (II.) relictum* ssp. *relictum* and *P. (N.) nucleophilum*.

Contents

1

Introduction

The huge and diversified avian fauna of Southeast Asia was summarized by King and Dickinson (1975) as numbering "1198 species that are known to have occurred prior to 31 May 1971 in Burma, Malaya, Thailand, Indochina (Laos, Cambodia, and Vietnam) and Hong Kong". By 1975, Malaya had already become Malaysia, Burma has since become Myanmar, and Indochina is seldom heard nowadays. Meanwhile, war and economic factors in the region have caused great destruction of rainforests. The resultant habitat depletion has led to major reductions of populations for many species of birds and the extinction of others.

It was therefore most fortunate for the recording of the then-presence in the Asian Tropical Subregion of true malaria parasites of birds (Kingdom Protista: Phylum Apicomplexa: Family Plasmodiidae: Genus *Plasmodium*), that the project called the Migratory Animal Pathological Survey (MAPS) took place between 1963 and 1971. This came into being after the United States Army's 406th Medical General Laboratory had collected peripheral blood films from birds in Honshu, Japan, during the 1950s; being followed by the United States Army Medical Research (USAMR) Unit's further studies from the Institute of Medical Research (IMR) at Kuala Lumpur (capital of Malaysia). From 1954 to 1957 the author was on the faculty of the University of Malaya (now the National University of Singapore). He received USAMR/IMR material from Dr. H. Elliott McClure, and as a consequence published (Laird 1962) the first accounts of *Plasmodium vaughani* and *P. rouxi* from Malaysia. Unfortunately though, his manuscript reviewing the avian haematozoa identified for USAMR/IMR was "lost at the Raffles Museum in Singapore when the publication of the Raffles Bulletin was discontinued" (McClure *et al.* 1978).

Soon afterwards Dr. McClure assumed the leadership of MAPS, and from 1963 the author (then in a purely administrative World Health Organization (WHO) Secretariat post in Geneva) received increasing quantities of avian blood smears from the MAPS project based initially at Kuala Lumpur and then at Bangkok, Thailand. The MAPS sampling area duly extended to much of the Asian Tropical Subregion[1] and its western (Iranian) and eastern (Japanese) bordering zones.

[1] The zoogeographical scheme followed herein is that of Darlington (1957) as presented by Neill (1969).

On the author's return to academic life at Canada's Memorial University of Newfoundland (MUN), the by-then very considerable collection of MAPS blood smears became the basis for what was first designated the WHO International Reference Centre for Avian Malaria Parasites, and afterwards the International Reference Centre for Avian Haematozoa (IRCAH) (McClure *et al.* 1978). McClure *et al.* published a preliminary overview of the MAPS material. With the exception of some species of *Plasmodium*, none of the identifications in that account were taken beyond the genus level. MUN/IRCAH has recently been disbanded, and its collections transferred to the Queensland Museum, South Brisbane, Australia.

2

Methods and material

More than 99% of all birds handled by MAPS were mist-netted, leg-banded and released after toenail clipping to obtain the necessary drop of peripheral blood for a thin smear. The remainder were purchased from local collectors who captured them for use as food, or in relatively few cases, shot the birds. When dry, the smears were methanol fixed, and sent to MAPS headquarters for Giemsa staining. Consignments were initially sent to the author's home in Switzerland by sea freight (water damage en route sometimes necessitating time-consuming salvage, relabelling, etc.; see Figure 2.1). Later consignments went directly to the International Reference Centre in St John's, Newfoundland.

Following receipt, each smear was scanned microscopically after covering with a thin film of immersion oil, first under a low-power dry objective to detect microfilariae. An oil immersion objective was then used in a 20 min search for other haematozoa. Until the establishment of the WHO International Reference Centre for Avian Malaria Parasites in 1968 (Bennett and Laird 1971), the author reported identifications to the genus level (except in the case of microfilariae) to MAPS for their guidance as to possible vectors that might also be implicated in arbovirus transmission to humans from avian transport hosts.

A decade later McClure *et al.* (1978) were able to list the following positives from the then-accessioned smears from 55 289 birds, of 1132 species:

Table 2.1 Number of positives from smears (McClure *et al.* 1978)

	No. of smears	%
Total +ve for haematozoa	9026	16.3
+ve for *Haemoproteus*	6256	11.3
+ve for *Leucocytozoon*	1478	2.7
+ve for microfilariae	1011	1.8
+ve for minor taxa	616	1.1
+ve for *Plasmodium*	422	0.8
+ve for *Trypanosoma*	114	0.2

Many valuable publications on most of these taxa have now resulted from the investigations of Prof. G. F. Bennett (who assumed responsibility for the International Reference Centre when the author became Director of Memorial's Research Unit on Vector Pathology in 1973) and his students and colleagues. However, the author, whose personal interest was in the *Plasmodium* slides, retained these for later study. Shortly before his retirement to New Zealand in 1983, at which stage the Giemsa stain of many (particularly those from earlier consignments that had suffered in-transit damage as earlier mentioned) was noticeably fading, he spent many weeks re-examining these slides, and photographing hundreds of the best examples of the various malaria parasites by means of a Zeiss Axiomat. The former incorporated fully automatic camera facilities. Polaroid ASA400 monochrome film was used. Very accurate measurements were subsequently made from the resultant prints, thanks to the incorporated scale-line synchronized with the microscope's zoom lens system.

In the course of that microscopy and the final months of re-examination while preparing this paper, further mixed infections of *Plasmodium* spp. were recognized, and errors were found in the McClure *et al.* (1978) malaria-positive birds count. The final such figure for the MAPS collections is 536, or 0.97% of the overall total of 55 289 birds sampled and 2.03% of the 26 385 birds of malarious species (Table 2.2).

Of the 1132 avian species studied, 180 (15.9%) harboured *Plasmodium*. Appendix A of McClure *et al.* (1978) lists the families and scientific names of all 1132. These authors also provide common names for all species harbouring haematozoa. Their nomenclature accords with then-current checklists, family order following Austin (1961) and English vernacular names, Edwards (1974). Only the *Plasmodium*-positive species are listed in Table 2.2, in accordance with the radically new classification of birds based upon DNA-DNA hybridization studies (Sibley *et al.* 1988; Sibley and Monroe 1990); except that for ease of reference all genera and species are presented alphabetically. Italicized names within square brackets between some generic and specific names are the senior ones of relevant superspecies, while numbers within square brackets following English common names are those of the World List numbering system (Sibley and Monroe 1990).

Table 2.2 List of the birds harbouring *Plasmodium*

	No. of birds	No. +ve *Plasmodium*
Class AVES		
Subclass NEORNITHES		
Infraclass NEOAVES		
Parvclass GALOANSERAE		
Superorder GALLOMORPHAE		
Order **GALLIFORMES**		
Parvorder PHASIANIDA		
Superfamily PHASIANOIDEA		
Family **Phasianidae** (Grouse, Pheasants, etc.)		
Argusianus [argus] argus (Linnaeus) 1766		
Great Argus [3109]	3	1

Table 2.2 (*cont.*)

	No. of birds	No. +ve *Plasmodium*
Coturnix [chinensis] chinensis (Linnaeus) 1766		
Blue-breasted Quail [3061]	197	5
Gallus [gallus] gallus (Linnaeus) 1758		
Red Junglefowl [309.4]	17	1
Lophura erythropthalma (Raffles) 1822		
Crestless Fireback [3092]	8	1
Superorder ANSERIMORPHAE		
Order **ANSERIFORMES**		
Infraorder ANSERIDES		
Family **Anatidae**		
Subfamily Anatinae		
Tribe Anserini (Geese)		
Anser anser Linnaeus 1758		
Greylag Goose [2060]	28	1
Tribe Anatini (Typical Ducks)		
Netta rufina (Pallas) 1773		
Red-crested Pochard [145]	32	1
Parvclass TURNICAE		
Order **TURNICIFORMES**		
Family **Turnicidae** (Buttonquails)		
Turnix suscitator (Gmelin) 1789		
Barred Buttonquail [2178]	141	8
Parvclass PICAE		
Order **PICIFORMES**		
Infraorder PICIDES		
Family **Picidae** (Woodpeckers, Wrynecks)		
Dryocopus [javensis] javensis (Horsfield) 1821		
White-bellied Woodpecker [2394]	3	1
Infraorder RAMPHASTIDES		
Superfamily MEGALAIMOIDEA		
Family **Megalaimidae** (Asian Barbets)		
Megalaima [asiatica] asiatica (Latham) 1790		
Blue-throated Barbet [3366]	25	1
Megalaima chrysopogon (Temminck) 1824		
Gold-whiskered Barbet [3359]	1	1
Megalaima faiostricta (Temminck) 1831		
Green-eared Barbet [3357]	6	2
Megalaima mystacophanos (Temminck) 1824		
Red-throated Barbet [3361]	7	1
Parvclass CORACIAE		
Superorder BUCEROTIMORPHAE		
Order **UPUPIFORMES**		
Infraorder UPUPIDES		
Family **Upupidae** (Hoopoes)		
Upupa [epops] epops (Linnaeus) 1758		
Eurasian Hoopoe [391.1]	91	4

Table 2.2 (*cont.*)

	No. of birds	No. +ve *Plasmodium*
Superorder CORACIIMORPHAE		
Order **CORACIIFORMES**		
Suborder ALCEDINI		
Infraorder ALCEDINIDES		
Parvorder CERYLIDA		
Superfamily DACELONOIDEA		
Family **Dacelonidae** (Dacelonid Kingfishers)		
Halcyon pileata (Boddaert) 1783		
Black-capped Kingfisher [2364]	179	1
Todirhamphus [chloris] chloris (Boddaert) 1783		
Collared Kingfisher [2366]	596	1
Infraorder MEROPIDES		
Family **Meropidae** (Bee-eaters)		
Merops orientalis Latham 1801		
Little Green Bee-eater [2355]	115	3
Parvclass PASSERAE		
Superorder CUCULIMORPHAE		
Order **CUCULIFORMES**		
Infraorder CUCULIDES		
Parvorder CUCULIDA		
Superfamily CUCULOIDEA		
Family **Cuculidae** (Old World Cuckoos)		
Cuculus [canorus] canorus Linnaeus 1758		
Common Cuckoo [388.2]	31	1
Eudynamys [scolopacea] scolopacea (Linnaeus) 1758		
Asian Koel [3217]	60	1
Phaenicophaeus javanicus Horsfield 1821		
Red-billed Malkoha [3224]	2	2
Superfamily CENTROPODOIDEA		
Family **Centropodidae** (Coucals)		
Centropus [sinensis] sinensis (Stephens) 1815		
Greater Coucal [3234]	28	1
Superorder PSITTACIMORPHAE		
Order **PSITTACIFORMES**		
Family **Psittacidae** (Parrots, Macaws, etc.)		
Loriculus galgulus (Linnaeus) 1758		
Blue-crowned Hanging-Parrot [3199]	5	2
Prioniturus [discurus] discurus (Vieillot) 1822		
Blue-crowned Racquet-tail [3101]	8	1
Prioniturus [platenae] platenae Blasius 1888		
Blue-headed Racquet-tail [3192.1]	12	1
Trichoglossus [haematodus] haematodus (Linnaeus) 1771		
Rainbow Lorikeet [3184]	1	1

Table 2.2 (*cont.*)

	No. of birds	No. +ve *Plasmodium*
Superorder STRIGIMORPHAE		
Order **STRIGIFORMES**		
Suborder STRIGI		
Parvorder TYTONIDA		
Family **Tytonidae** (Barn and Grass Owls)		
Phodilus badius (Horsfield) 1821		
Oriental Bay-Owl [3241]	15	1
Parvorder STRIGIDA		
Family **Strigidae** (Typical Owls)		
Athene brama (Temminck) 1821		
Spotted Owlet [2326]	31	5
Glaucidium [castanopterum] cuculoides (Vigors) 1831		
Asian Barred Owlet [3257]	14	2
Ninox philippensis Bonaparte 1855		
Philippine Hawk-Owl [3259]	49	2
Ninox scutulata (Raffles) 1822		
Brown Hawk-Owl [2324]	47	2
Otus [bakkamoena] lempiji (Horsfield) 1821		
Collared Scops-Owl [2314.2]	229	10
Otus [spilocephalus][1] *spilocephalus* (Blyth) 1846		
Mountain Scops-Owl [3244]	42	3
Otus [scops] sunia (Hodgson) 1836		
Oriental Scops-Owl [374.1]	102	3
Superorder PASSERIMORPHAE		
Order **COLUMBIFORMES**		
Family **Columbidae** (Pigeons, Doves)		
Chalcophaps indica (Linnaeus) 1758		
Emerald Dove [2294]	629	3
Phapitreron leucotis (Temminck) 1823		
White-eared Brown-Dove [3152]	142	1
Streptopelia chinensis (Scopoli) 1786		
Spotted Dove [315.1]	103	4
Treron [curvirostra] curvirostra (Gmelin) 1789		
Thick-billed Green-Pigeon [3159]	40	1
Treron sphenura (Vigors) 1832		
Wedge-tailed Green-Pigeon [2296]	3	1
Order **GRUIFORMES**		
Suborder RALLI		
Family **Rallidae** (Rails, Gallinules and Coots)		
Amaurornis phoenicurus (Pennant) 1769		
White-breasted Waterhen [2191]	79	23
Porzana cinerea (Vieillot) 1819		
White-browed Crake [2186]	97	1
Rallina eurizonoides (Lafresnaye) 1845		
Slaty-legged Crake [2181]	120	6

[1] Within genera alphabetical order is by species-name, not the relevant superspecies one.

Table 2.2 (*cont.*)

	No. of birds	No. +ve *Plasmodium*
Rallina fasciata (Raffles) 1822		
Red-legged Crake [3112]	7	1
Order **CICONIIFORMES**		
Suborder CHARADRII		
Infraorder CHARADRIIDES		
Parvorder SCOLOPACIDA		
Superfamily SCOLOPACOIDEA		
Family **Scolopacidae**		
Subfamily Tringinae (Sandpipers, Curlews, Phalaropes)		
Tringa glareola Linnaeus 1758		
Wood Sandpiper [257.1]	265	1
Tringa hypoleucos Linnaeus 1758		
Common Sandpiper [263.1]	262	1
Superfamily JACONOIDEA		
Family **Rostratulidae** (Painted-snipe)		
Rostratula [benghalensis] benghalensis (Linnaeus) 1758		
Greater Painted-snipe [2233]	182	1
Suborder CICONII		
Infraorder FALCONIDES		
Parvorder ACCIPITRIDA		
Family **Accipitridae**		
Subfamily Accipitrinae (Hawks, Eagles)		
Accipiter [badius] badius (Gmelin 1788)		
Shikra [2102]	30	1
Accipiter [virgatus] virgatus (Temminck) 1822		
Besra [3035.2]	71	1
Sarcogyps calvus (Scopoli) 1786		
Red-headed Vulture [3032]	1	1
Infraorder CICONIIDES		
Parvorder CICONIIDA		
Superfamily ARDEOIDEA		
Family **Ardeidae** (Herons, Bitterns, Egrets)		
Butorides [striatus] striatus (Linnaeus) 1758		
Striated Heron [1014.1]	50	2
Ixobrychus cinnamomeus (Gmelin) 1789		
Cinnamon Bittern [2029]	197	3
Ixobrychus [minutus] sinensis (Gmelin) 1789		
Yellow Bittern [2027]	75	2
Order **PASSERIFORMES**		
Suborder TYRANNI		
Infraorder EURYLAIMIDES		
Superfamily PITTOIDEA		
Family **Pittidae** (Pittas)		
Pitta [brachyura] brachyura (Linnaeus) 1766		
Indian Pitta [3435.1]	29	2

Table 2.2 (*cont.*)

	No. of birds	No. +ve *Plasmodium*
Pitta [erythrogaster] erythrogaster Temminck 1823		
Red-bellied Pitta [3431]	143	3
Pitta [brachyura] moluccensis (Müller) 1776		
Blue-winged Pitta [3437]	58	2
Pitta phayrei (Blyth) 1863		
Eared Pitta [3420]	3	1
Suborder PASSERI		
Parvorder CORVIDA		
Superfamily CORVOIDEA		
Family **Irenidae** (Fairy-bluebirds, Leafbirds)		
Chloropsis cyanopogon (Temminck) 1829		
Lesser Green Leafbird [3576]	8	1
Family **Laniidae** (True Shrikes)		
Lanius collurioides Lesson 1834		
Burmese Shrike [3875]	8	2
Lanius [cristatus] cristatus Linnaeus 1758		
Brown Shrike [621.1]	719	57
Lanius schach Linnaeus 1758[2]		
Long-tailed Shrike [2849]	130	15
Lanius validirostris Ogilvie-Grant 1894		
Mountain Shrike [3876]	2	2
Family **Corvidae**		
Subfamily Pachycephalinae		
Tribe Pachycephalini (Whistlers, Shrike-thrushes)		
Pachycephala [grisola] grisola (Blyth) 1843		
Mangrove Whistler [3678]	129	1
Subfamily Corvinae		
Tribe Corvini (Crows, Magpies, Jays, Nutcrackers)		
Dendrocitta vagabunda (Latham) 1790		
Rufous Treepie [3452]	35	1
Tribe Oriolini (Orioles, Cuckooshrikes)		
Oriolus [chinensis] chinensis Linnaeus 1766		
Black-naped Oriole [2460]	219	4
Pericrocotus [roseus] divaricatus (Raffles) 1822		
Ashy Minivet [2510]	7	1
Subfamily Dicrurinae		
Tribe Rhipidurini (Fantails) (Vieillot) 1818		
Rhipidura albicollis ¶[3] *albogularis* (Lesson) 1832		
Spot-breasted Fantail [3672.1]	12	1
Rhipidura javanica (Sparrman) 1788		
Pied Fantail [3675]	813	2
Tribe Dicrurini (Drongos)		
Dicrurus annectans (Hodgson) 1836		
Crow-billed Drongo [3465]	30	2

[2] Including *L. nasutus* (Scopoli) as presented in McClure *et al.* (1978) — this specific designation is reduced to a group name within *L. schach* by Sibley and Monroe (1990).

[3] The symbol ¶ precedes group names herein, in accordance with Sibley and Monroe (1990).

Table 2.2 (*cont.*)

	No. of birds	No. +ve *Plasmodium*
Dicrurus [balicassius] balicassius (Linnaeus) 1766		
Balicassiao [3468]	80	3
Dicrurus hottentottus (Linnaeus) 1766		
Hair-crested Drongo [2458]	93	5
Dicrurus [adsimilis] macrocercus (Vieillot) 1817		
Black Drongo [2456]	115	1
Dicrurus paradiseus (Linnaeus) 1766		
Greater Racket-tailed Drongo [3470]	104	1
Dicrurus remifer (Temminck) 1823		
Lesser Racket-tailed Drongo [3467]	170	1
Tribe Monarchini (Monarchs, Magpie-larks)		
Hypothymis azurea (Boddaert) 1783		
Black-naped Monarch [3664]	204	1
Tersiphone [cinnamomea] cyanescens (Sharpe) 1877		
Blue Paradise-Flycatcher [3667]	32	1
Subfamily Malaconotinae		
Tribe Vangini (Helmet-shrikes, Vangas)		
Tephrodornis gularis (Raffles) 1822		
Large Woodshrike [3520]	23	1
Parvorder PASSERIDA		
Superfamily MUSCICAPOIDEA		
Family **Muscicapidae**		
Subfamily Turdinae (True Thrushes)		
Turdus cardis Temminck 1831		
Japanese Thrush [2727]	28	2
Turdus [pallidus] chrysolaus Temminck 1831		
Brown-headed Thrush [2732]	43	1
Turdus [unicolor] hortulorum Sclater 1863		
Grey-backed Thrush [2735]	32	1
Turdus obscurus Gmelin 1789		
Eyebrowed Thrush [761.3]	260	5
Turdus [pallidus] pallidus Gmelin 1789		
Pale Thrush [2736]	48	1
Zoothera cinerea (Bourns and Worcester) 1894		
Ashy Thrush [3718]	51	1
Zoothera citrina (Latham) 1790		
Orange-headed Thrush [3719]	124	1
Zoothera marginata Blyth 1847		
Dark-sided Thrush [3715]	10	1
Zoothera sibirica (Pallas) 1776		
Siberian Thrush [2745]	104	10
Subfamily Muscicapinae		
Tribe Muscicapini (Old World Flycatchers)		
Cyanoptila cyanomelana (Temminck) 1829		
Blue-and-white Flycatcher [2641]	26	1
Ficedula [narcissina] narcissina (Temminck) 1835		
Narcissus Flycatcher [2632]	60	1

Table 2.2 (*cont.*)

	No. of birds	No. +ve *Plasmodium*
Niltava grandis (Blyth) 1842		
Large Niltava [2636]	129	1
Tribe Saxicolini (Chats)		
Copsychus malabaricus (Scopoli) 1788		
White-rumped Shama [769]	288	13
Copsychus [niger] niger (Sharpe) 1877		
White-vented Shama [3688]	31	2
Copsychus [saularis] saularis (Linnaeus) 1758		
Oriental Magpie-Robin [3685]	862	22
Enicurus ruficapillus Temminck 1823		
Chestnut-naped Forktail [3698]	30	1
Enicurus schistaceus (Hodgson) 1836		
Slaty-backed Forktail [2715]	27	1
Luscinia cyane (Pallas) 1776		
Siberian Blue Robin [764.3]	315	5
Phoenicurus auroreus (Pallas) 1776		
Daurian Redstart [2683]	50	1
Saxicola caprata (Linnaeus) 1766		
Pied Bushchat [2711]	73	1
Saxicoloides fulicata (Linnaeus) 1766		
Indian Robin [2689]	61	2
Family **Sturnidae**		
Tribe Sturnini (Starlings, Mynas)		
Acridotheres [javanicus] grandis Moore 1858		
White-vented Myna [3890]	115	1
Acridotheres tristis (Linnaeus) 1766		
Common Myna [493.2]	125	4
Ampeliceps coronatus Blyth 1842		
Golden-crested Myna [3892]	15	1
Aplonis panayensis (Scopoli) 1783		
Asian Glossy Starling [3879]	259	2
Sarcops calvus (Linnaeus) 1766		
Coleto [3894]	130	3
Sturnus contra Linnaeus 1758		
Asian Pied Starling [3884]	194	4
Sturnus malabaricus (Gmelin) 1789		
Chestnut-tailed Starling [3882]	47	2
Sturnus nigricollis (Paykull) 1807		
Black-collared Starling [3885]	110	6
Superfamily SYLVIOIDEA		
Family **Sittidae**		
Subfamily Sittinae (Nuthatches)		
Sitta azurea Lesson 1830		
Blue Nuthatch [3493]	3	1
Family **Paridae**		
Subfamily Parinae (Titmice, Chickadees)		
Parus [xanthogenys] xanthogenys Vigors 1831		
Black-lored Tit [3484]	30	1

Table 2.2 (*cont.*)

	No. of birds	No. +ve *Plasmodium*
Family **Pycnonotidae** (Bulbuls)		
Hypsipetes [madagascariensis] leucocephalus (Gmelin) 1789		
Black Bulbul [3567.1]	46	3
Iole olivacea Blyth 1844		
Buff-vented Bulbul [3557]	8	1
Ixos amaurotis (Temminck) 1830		
Brown-eared Bulbul [2520]	28	1
Ixos [philippinus] philippinus (Forster) 1795		
Philippine Bulbul [3560]	402	1
Pycnonotus blanfordi Jerdon 1862		
Streak-eared Bulbul [3544]	973	25
Pycnonotus brunneus Blyth 1845		
Red-eyed Bulbul [3546]	80	1
Pycnonotus [cafer] cafer (Linnaeus) 1766		
Red-vented Bulbul [726.2]	230	6
Pycnonotus erythropthalmos (Hume) 1878		
Spectacled Bulbul [3547]	46	2
Pycnonotus finlaysoni Strickland 1844		
Stripe-throated Bulbul [3537]	184	4
Pycnonotus flavescens Blyth 1845		
Flavescent Bulbul [3540)]	183	1
Pycnonotus [goiavier] goiavier (Scopoli) 1786		
Yellow-vented Bulbul [3541]	2602	7
Pycnonotus jocosus (Linnaeus) 1758		
Red-whiskered Bulbul [726.1]	202	3
Pycnonotus [cafer] leucogenys (Gray) 1835		
Himalayan Bulbul [2516]	48	3
Pycnonotus melanicterus (Gmelin) 1789		
Black-crested Bulbul [3529]	198	13
Pycnonotus melanoleucos (Eyton) 1839		
Black-and-white Bulbul [3526]	5	4
Pycnonotus plumosus Blyth 1845		
Olive-winged Bulbul [3543]	1339	3
Pycnonotus simplex Lesson 1839		
Cream-vented Bulbul [3545]	99	1
Pycnonotus sinensis (Gmelin) 1789		
Light-vented Bulbul [2515]	121	1
Pycnonotus squamatus (Temminck) 1828		
Scaly-breasted Bulbul [3530]	1	1
Family **Cisticolidae** (African Warblers)		
Prinia familiaris Horsfield 1821		
Bar-winged Prinia [3603]	48	1
Prinia flaviventris (Delessert) 1840		
Yellow-bellied Prinia [3604]	99	2
Prinia hodgsonii Blyth 1844		
Grey-breasted Prinia [3601]	50	1
Prinia [subflava] inornata Sykes 1832		
Plain Prinia [2541]	74	1

Table 2.2 (*cont.*)

	No. of birds	No. +ve *Plasmodium*
Prinia socialis Sykes 1832		
Ashy Prinia [3605]	42	1
Family **Zosteropidae** (White-eyes)		
Zosterops [palpebrosus] japonicus Temminck and Schlegel 1847		
Japanese White-eye [622.6]	149	1
Zosterops [palpebrosus] palpebrosus (Temminck) 1824		
Oriental White-eye [2868]	165	6
Family **Sylviidae**		
Subfamily Acrocephalinae (Leaf-Warblers)		
Acrocephalus aedon (Pallas) 1776		
Thick-billed Warbler [2565]	106	3
Acrocephalus [arundinaceus] orientalis (Temminck and Schlegel) 1847		
Oriental Reed-Warbler [2564.1]	566	2
Acrocephalus [arundinaceus] stentoreus (Ehrenberg) 1833		
Clamorous Reed-Warbler [2563]	85	1
Hippolais caligata (Lichtenstein) 1823		
Booted Warbler [2567]	14	1
Locustella [fasciolata] fasciolata (Gray) 1860		
Gray's Warbler [2550]	44	3
Locustella lanceolata (Temminck) 1840		
Lanceolated Warbler [747.5]	166	1
Orthotomus sutorius (Pennant) 1769		
Common Tailorbird [3607]	249	1
Subfamily Garrulacinae (Laughingthrushes)		
Garrulax [erythrocephalus] erythrocephalus (Vigors) 1832		
Chestnut-crowned Laughingthrush [2778]	141	1
Garrulax lineatus (Vigors) 1831		
Streaked Laughingthrush [2773]	9	2
Subfamily Sylviinae		
Tribe Timaliini (Babblers)		
Alcippe peracensis Sharpe 1887		
Mountain Fulvetta [3852]	162	1
Alcippe poioicephala (Jerdon) 1844		
Brown-cheeked Fulvetta [3850]	162	1
Chrysomma sinense (Gmelin) 1789		
Yellow-eyed Babbler [3803]	82	1
Heterophasia melanoleuca (Blyth) 1859		
Black-headed Sibia [3858]	128	1
Macronous gularis (Horsfield) 1822		
Striped Tit-Babbler [3797]	409	1
Minla strigula (Hodgson) 1837		
Chestnut-tailed Minla [2787]	164	3
Pellorneum ruficeps Swainson 1832		
Puff-throated Babbler [3722]	198	1

Table 2.2 (*cont.*)

	No. of birds	No. +ve *Plasmodium*
Pomatorhinus hypoleucos (Blyth) 1844		
Large Scimitar-Babbler [3743]	7	1
Pomatorhinus ruficollis Hodgson 1836		
Streak-breasted Scimitar-Babbler [2547]	21	1
Pomatorhinus [horsfieldii] schisticeps Hodgson 1836		
White-browed Scimitar-Babbler [3745]	138	2
Pteruthius flaviscapis (Temminck) 1835		
White-browned Shrike-Babbler [2783]	7	1
Stachyris poliocephala (Temminck) 1836		
Grey-headed Babbler [3785]	88	5
Trichastoma rostratum (Blyth) 1842		
White-chested Babbler [3731]	242	17
Yuhina zantholeuca (Blyth) 1844		
White-bellied Yuhina [3866]	58	3
Tribe Sylviini (*Sylvia*)		
Sylvia curruca ¶ *curruca* (Linnaeus) 1758		
Lesser Whitethroat [2585]	90	1
Superfamily PASSEROIDEA		
Family **Alaudidae** (Larks)		
Galerida cristata (Linnaeus) 1758		
Crested Lark [2416]	27	1
Mirafra assamica Horsfield 1840		
Rufous-winged Lark [3438]	47	1
Family **Nectariniidae**		
Subfamily Nectariniinae		
Tribe Dicaeini (Flowerpeckers)		
Dicaeum [cruentatum] cruentatum (Linnaeus) 1758		
Scarlet-backed Flowerpecker [3932]	66	1
Tribe Nectariniini (Sunbirds, Spiderhunters)		
Aethopyga shelleyi Sharpe 1876		
Lovely Sunbird [3951]	8	1
Anthreptes malacensis (Scopoli) 1786		
Plain-throated Sunbird [3937]	913	3
Arachnothera magna (Hodgson) 1837		
Streaked Spiderhunter [3964]	55	1
Nectarinia [asiatica] asiatica (Latham) 1790		
Purple Sunbird [2875]	72	2
Nectarinia jugularis (Linnaeus) 1776		
Olive-backed Sunbird [3946]	128	5
Nectarinia [sperata] sperata (Linnaeus) 1766		
Purple-throated Sunbird [3943]	8	1
Nectarinia zeylonica (Linnaeus) 1766		
Purple-rumped sunbird [3941]	30	1
Family **Passeridae**		
Subfamily Passerinae (Sparrows, Rock Sparrows, etc.)		
Passer domesticus (Linnaeus) 1758		
House Sparrow [688.2]	127	7
Passer flaveolus (Blyth) 1844		
Plain-backed Sparrow [3968]	345	4

Table 2.2 (*cont.*)

		No. of birds	No. +ve *Plasmodium*
	Subfamily Motacillinae (Wagtails, Pipits)		
	Anthus hodgsoni (Richmond) 1907		
	Olive-backed Pipit [698.3]	290	1
	Motacilla [alba] alba (Linnaeus) 1758		
	White Wagtail [694]	214	1
	Subfamily Ploceinae (Weavers)		
	Ploceus manyar (Horsfield) 1821		
	Streaked Weaver [2989]	66	1
	Ploceus philippinus (Linnaeus) 1766		
	Baya Weaver [2971]	462	10
	Subfamily Estrildinae		
	Tribe Estrildini (Waxbills, Estrildines)		
	Erythrura [prasina] prasina (Sparrman) 1788		
	Pin-tailed Parrotfinch [3975]	40	1
	Lonchura maja (Linnaeus) 1766		
	White-headed Munia [3983]	39	1
	Lonchura [malacca] malacca (Linnaeus) 1766		
	Black-headed Munia [812]	299	4
	Lonchura punctulata (Linnaeus) 1758		
	Scaly-breasted Munia [811]	349	1
	Family **Fringillidae**		
	Subfamily Emberizinae		
	Tribe Emberizini (Buntings, Longspurs, Towhees)		
	Emberiza aureola Pallas 1773		
	Yellow-breasted Bunting [535.6]	230	2
	Emberiza cioides (Brandt) 1843		
	Meadow Bunting [2886]	98	1
	Emberiza elegans Temminck 1835		
	Yellow-throated Bunting [2900]	121	1
	Emberiza fucata Pallas 1776		
	Chestnut-eared Bunting [2898]	79	1
	Emberiza rutila Pallas 1776		
	Chestnut Bunting [2902]	390	1
Totals	180 species of 35 families	26 385	538

The following table summarizes data for locating the various collections of *Plasmodium*-infected birds. It includes many little-known places. From his own exhaustive notes, Dr. H. Elliott McClure was only unable to place one of them. Map coordinates are listed in Table 2.3.

Table 2.3 Map coordinates of collection data

Bhutan:	27.00N × 91.00E.
China:	Hong Kong, 22.30N × 114.00E.
India:	Gujurat, 23.00N × 71.00E; Kashmir, 34.00N × 74.00E; Kutch, 23.30N × 70.00E; Mahabaleshwar, Maharashtra, 17.56N ×

	73.42E; Orissa, 20.00N × 85.00E; Rajasthan, 27.00N × 77.00E; Tamil Nadu, 10.00N × 80.00E.
Indonesia:	Bali, 8.10S × 114.30E.
Iran:	Mahárlú, 29.36N × 52.53E.
Japan:	Tsunoshima, Yamaguchi, 34.21N × 130.51E; Shinhama, Ichikawa, Chiba, 35.40N × 139.55E.
Malaysia (W):	Bukit Besi, 4.46N × 103.12E; Gombak, Selangor, 3.21N × 101.47E; Kuala Kangsar, 4.50N × 100.55E; Kuala Lumpur, 3.08N × 101.42E; Mt Brinchang, Cameron Heights, Pahang, 4.31N × 101.25E; Muar, Johore, 2.01N × 102.35E; Rantau Panjang, Selangor, 03.05N × 101.24E; Subang, Johore 2.45N × 102.42E; Sungei Way, Selangor, 3.12N × 101.40E.
Malaysia (E):	Kuching, Sarawak, 1.30N × 110.20E; Pandan, Sarawak, 3.14N × 113.26E; Tuaran, Sabah, 6.12N × 116.12E.
Philippines:	Aborlan, Palawan, 9.20N × 118.20E; Basay, Negros Oriental, 9.27N × 122.38E; Batangas, Calatagan, Luzon, 13.48N × 120.37E; Bayawan, Negros Oriental, 9.21N × 122.47E; Camarines Norte, Luzon, 14.05N × 122.55E; Dalton Pass, Nueva Vizcaya, Luzon, 16.08N × 120.55E; Iwahig, Palawan, 9.40N × 118.27E; Lanao del Norte, Mindanao, 8.00N × 124.00E; Panagturan Point, Palawan, 9.41N × 118.45E; Pasi, Mindoro Oriental, 13.07N × 121.18E; Siaton, Negros Oriental, 8.55N × 123.00E; Puerto Princessa, Palawan, 9.40N × 118.40E; Tarabanan, Palawan (unlocated).
South Korea:	Chinchup-Myun, 37.45N × 127.15E.
Taiwan:	Ping-tung, 22.40N × 120.30E.
Thailand:	Ban Chiang Dao, 19.22N × 98.59E; Bangkok, 13.44N × 100.30E; Bang Phra, Cholburi, 13.12N × 100.50E; Chanthaburi, 12.35N × 102.08E; Chiang Mai, 18.48N × 98.58E; Koh Kred, Pak Kred, Nakhon Ratchasima, 15.00N × 102.06E; Ranong, 9.58N × 98.35E; Sakaerat, Pakthong Chai, 14.30N × 101.56E; Sara Buri, 14.32N × 100.53E.

3

Genus-level identifications of Plasmodium

Of the 538 individual birds harbouring *Plasmodium*, the 257 (47.8%) for which neither specific nor subgeneric identification of their parasites was feasible, are listed in Table 3.1, together with data concerning any associated haematozoa, localities and months of collection. Sometimes failure to go beyond the generic level reflected poor smearing or fixing under humid field conditions, imperfect staining, damage in transit (Figure 2.1) or subsequent fading. While in mixed infections occasional confusion was caused by multiple invasions of red cells (Figure 3.1) rendering subgeneric identification difficult, very low parasitaemias were the usual cause of inability to venture more than "*Plasmodium* sp?". Also in the Asian Tropical Subregion, such experienced investigators as Manwell, Allen and Kuntz (1976) had been unable to identify the specific malarias of 40 (51.3%) of the *Plasmodium* hosts among 1477 Taiwanese birds examined. They stated that this was "Because often only 1 or 2 parasites were seen on a slide". This and the approximately 50% incidence of generic identifications only, accorded remarkably closely with lengthy personal experience with MAPS material. Figure 3.2 illustrates the only *Plasmodium* discovered after a methodical 1 h 5 min search of a *Trichastoma rostratum* slide from Malaysia, previously searched by the author and others on three occasions without any more than a "*Plasmodium?*" finding. Unsupported by other life-history stages, this polar schizont tempted a guess at some species of the subgenus *Giovannolaia*. Without supporting evidence though, such a diagnosis was inadmissible — despite the fact that the same host yielded two species of this subgenus on other occasions at the same Malaysian locality, Rantau Panjang (see Tables 6.4 and 6.5).

Table 3.1 Findings of ***Plasmodium*** sp?

Host species[1]	Numbers recorded	Associated haematozoa[2]	Localities	Months
Coturnix chinensis	1	*H*	Palawan, Philippines	March
Coturnix chinensis	1	–	Palawan, Philippines	March
Lophura erythropthalma	1	*P.l.*	Subang, Malaysia	October
Anser anser	1	*H*	Rajasthan, India	November
Netta rufina	1	*H*	Northern India	December
Turnix suscitator	2	–	Kuala Lumpur, Malaysia	October
Megalaima mystacophanos	1	–	Southern Thailand	April
Megalaima faiostricta	1	–	Northern India	September
Megalaima faiostricta	1	–	Central India	February
Upupa epops	4	–	Rajasthan, India	Jan., Sept., Oct.
Halcyon pileata	1	*H*	Central Thailand	March
Merops orientalis	3	–	Rajasthan, India	September
Merops orientalis	2	–	Northern Thailand	May
Cuculus canorus	1	*Ae*	Luzon, Philippines	March
Centropus sinensis	1	–	Rajasthan, India	September
Phodilus badius	1	–	Lowland Malaysia	March
Athene brama	1	*H*	Central Thailand	December
Glaucidium cuculoides	1	*H, L*, mf	Nakhon Ratchasima, Thailand	June
Otus lempiji	2	*H*	Chiang Mai, Thailand	September
Otus lempiji	2	*H*	Luzon and Negros, Philippines	April
Otus lempiji	1	*H*	Malaysia	July
Otus lempiji	1	–	Sabah, E. Malaysia	April
Otus sunia	1	–	Japan	May
Otus sunia	1	–	Malaysia	May
Streptopelia chinensis	1	–	Negros, Philippines	November
Treron curvirostra	1	–	Palawan, Philippines	February
Treron sphenura	1	–	Bhutan	October
Rallina eurizonoides	1	*H, L*	Dalton Pass, Luzon, Philippines	May
Rallina eurizonoides	1	*H*, mf	Dalton Pass, Luzon, Philippines	April
Rallina eurizonoides	1	*L*	Dalton Pass, Luzon, Philippines	August
Rallina eurizonoides	3	–	Dalton Pass, Luzon, Philippines	December
Tringa glareola	1	–	Palawan, Philippines	September
Tringa hypoleucos	1	mf	Palawan, Philippines	September
Rostratula benghalensis	1	–	Palawan, Philippines	October
Accipiter badius	1	–	Central Thailand	December
Accipiter virgatus	1	*H*	Negros, Philippines	February
Butorides striatus	1	*T, H*, mf	Negros, Philippines	October
Butorides striatus	1	–	Negros, Philippines	October
Ixobrychus sinensis	1	*L*	Luzon, Philippines	October
Pitta brachyura	1	mf	Maharashtra, India	June
Pitta erythrogaster	1	–	Luzon, Philippines	June
Pitta phayrei	1	–	Central Thailand	September
Lanius collurioides	2	–	Northern Thailand	Oct., Dec.
Lanius cristatus	1	–	Calatagan, Luzon, Philippines	October
Lanius cristatus	1	–	Negros Oriental, Philippines	September
Lanius cristatus	1	–	Palawan, Philippines	September
Lanius cristatus	23[3]			
Lanius schach ¶ nasutus	2	–	Negros, Philippines	April
Lanius schach ¶ nasutus	1	–	Luzon, Philippines	August

Table 3.1 *(cont.)*

Host species[1]	Numbers recorded	Associated haematozoa[2]	Localities	Months
Lanius schach ¶ *schach*	1	*H*	Kashmir, India	April
Lanius schach ¶ *schach*	4	–	Maharashtra, India	Apr., Jul., Aug.
Lanius schach ¶ *schach*	1	–	Rajasthan, India	December
Lanius schach ¶ *schach*	1	–	Lowland Malaysia	June
Dendrocitta vagabunda	1	–	Rajasthan, India	February
Oriolus chinensis	2	mf	Siaton, Negros, Philippines	January
Rhipidura albicollis ¶ *albogularis*	1	*H*	Maharashtra, India	July
Rhipidura javanica	2	–	Central Thailand	June, Dec.
Dicrurus hottentottus	2	–	Luzon, Philippines	Mar., Apr.
Dicrurus macrocercus	1	–	Southern Thailand	November
Dicrurus paradiseus	1	–	Central Thailand	April
Dicrurus remifer	1	–	Northern Thailand	May
Hypothymis azurea	1	–	Palawan, Philippines	April
Tersiphone cyanescens	1	–	Palawan, Philippines	January
Tephrodornis gularis	1	–	Orissa, India	April
Turdus hortulorum	1	–	Hong Kong	December
Turdus obscurus	1	*L*	Malaysia	December
Turdus obscurus	1	–	Central Thailand	January
Turdus pallidus	1	–	Japan	October
Zoothera cinerea	1	–	Luzon, Philippines	January
Zoothera cinerea	1	–	Northern Thailand	October
Zoothera marginata	1	*H, L*	Northern Thailand	May
Cyanoptila cyanomelana	1	*H*	Japan	April
Ficedula narcissina	1	–	Japan	May
Niltava grandis	1	*L*	Highland Malaysia	January
Copsychus malabaricus	2	mf	Lowland Malaysia	Feb., Aug.
Copsychus malabaricus	1	*H*	Southern Thailand	June
Copsychus niger	1	*H*	Palawan, Philippines	April
Copsychus saularis	2	*H*	Central Thailand	Apr., Aug.
Copsychus saularis	1	*H*	Lowland Malaysia	June
Copsychus saularis	8[3]	?	?	?
Enicurus ruficapillus	1	mf	Southern Thailand	May
Enicurus schistaceus	1	–	Highland Malaysia	February
Phoenicurus auroreus	1	–	Japan	October
Saxicola caprata	1	–	Rajasthan, India	March
Saxicoloides fulicata	2	–	Maharashtra, India	July
Acridotheres grandis	1	*H*	Central Thailand	August
Acridotheres tristis	1	–	Central Thailand	August
Acridotheres tristis	1	–	Kashmir, India	April
Acridotheres tristis	1	–	Rajasthan, India	February
Acridotheres tristis	1	–	Gujarat, India	September
Ampeliceps coronatus	1	*H*	Central Thailand	January
Aplonis panayensis	1	–	Central Thailand	September
Sarcops calvus	1	*H*	Siaton, Negros, Philippines	December
Sturnus contra	1	*H*	Rajasthan, India	March
Sturnus contra	1	–	Rajasthan, India	March
Sturnus contra	1	–	Bali, Indonesia	March
Sturnus contra	1	–	Indonesia	May

Table 3.1 *(cont.)*

Host species[1]	Numbers recorded	Associated haematozoa[2]	Localities	Months
Sturnus malabaricus	1	–	Central Thailand	January
Sturnus malabaricus	1	–	Tamil Nadu, India	November
Sturnus nigricollis	2	*H*	Central Thailand	Feb., Apr.
Sturnus nigricollis	2	–	Central Thailand	May
Sitta azurea	1	*H*	Highland Malaysia	November
Parus xanthogenys	1	–	Orissa, India	May
Hypsipetes leucocephalus	1	*T*	Maharashtra, India	May
Hypsipetes leucocephalus	1	*H*	Maharashtra, India	April
Iole olivacea	1	–	Tarabanan, Palawan, Philippines	May
Pycnonotus blanfordi	22[3]	?	Central Thailand	?
Pycnonotus brunneus	1	–	Lowland Malaysia	June
Pycnonotus cafer	1	*L*	Maharashtra, India	July
Pycnonotus cafer	1	–	Gujarat, India	August
Pycnonotus cafer	1	–	Malaysia	October
Pycnonotus erythropthalmos	1	*L*	Northern Thailand	December
Pycnonotus erythropthalmos	1	–	Southern Thailand	November
Pycnonotus finlaysoni	1	*L*	Northern Thailand	December
Pycnonotus finlaysoni	3	–	Central Thailand	September
Pycnonotus goiavier	1	*H*	Negros, Philippines	February
Pycnonotus goiavier	1	*L*	Central Thailand	October
Pycnonotus jocosus	1	–	Maharashtra, India	May
Pycnonotus jocosus	1	–	Central Thailand	March
Pycnonotus leucogenys	1	*T*	Gujarat, India	November
Pycnonotus leucogenys	1	–	Rajasthan, India	September
Pycnonotus melanicterus	2	*L*	Northern Thailand	June
Pycnonotus melanicterus	1	*H, L*	Northern Thailand	June
Pycnonotus melanicterus	1	–	Northern Thailand	June
Pycnonotus melanicterus	2	*H*	Central Thailand	January
Pycnonotus melanicterus	3	–	Central Thailand	Jan., Apr.
Pycnonotus melanicterus	1	*T*	Highland Malaysia	June
Pycnonotus melanicterus	1	–	Palawan, Philippines	September
Pycnonotus plumosus	1	–	Palawan, Philippines	September
Prinia flaviventris	1	–	Lowland Malaysia	April
Prinia hodgsonii	1	–	Northern Thailand	July
Prinia inornata	1	–	Rajasthan, India	January
Prinia socialis	1	*T*	Maharashtra, India	July
Zosterops japonicus	4	–	Kashmir, India	April
Zosterops japonicus	1	–	Northern Thailand	December
Acrocephalus orientalis	1	–	Hong Kong	May
Hippolais caligata	1	–	Gujarat, India	September
Locustella fasciolata	2	–	Luzon, Philippines	September
Garrulax erythrocephalus	1	–	Bhutan	October
Garrulax lineatus	2	–	Bhutan	October
Alcippe peracensis	1	–	Taiwan	September
Chrysomma sinense	1	*L*	Maharashtra, India	July
Macronous gularis	1	mf	Palawan, Philippines	April
Minla strigula	1	–	Highland Malaysia	November
Pellorneum ruficeps	1	–	Northern Thailand	September

Table 3.1 *(cont.)*

Host species[1]	Numbers recorded	Associated haematozoa[2]	Localities	Months
Pomatorhinus ruficollis	1	–	Taiwan	September
Trichastoma rostratum	2	*At*	Rantau Panjang, Malaysia	February
Sylvia curruca ¶ *curruca*	1	*H*	Tamil Nadu, India	October
Mirafra assamica	1	–	Northern Thailand	January
Arachnothera magna	1	–	Highland Malaysia	?
Nectarinia asiatica	1	–	Maharashtra, India	July
Nectarinia sperata	1	*H*	Central Thailand	August
Nectarinia zeylonica	1	–	Maharashtra, India	July
Passer domesticus	2	*H*	Iran	July
Passer domesticus	5	–	Iran	Jul., Aug., Oct.
Passer flaveolus	4	–	Central Thailand	Jul., Aug.
Anthus hodgsoni	1	–	Northern Thailand	?
Erythrura prasina	1	–	Central Thailand	May
Lonchura malacca	1	–	Negros, Philippines	March
Lonchura malacca	1	–	Camarines Norte, Luzon, Philippines	April
Lonchura malacca	1	–	Subang, Malaysia	November
Emberiza aureola	1	–	Central Thailand	October
Emberiza cioides	1	–	Chinchup-Myun, S. Korea	June
Totals 114 host species	257 individuals +ve *Plasmodium*			

[1] Taxonomic order as in Table 2.2.

[2] *Aegyptianella (Ae), Trypanosoma (T), Haemoproteus (H), Plasmodium lophurae (P.l.), Leucocytozoon (L), Atoxoplasma (At)* and microfilariae (mf).

[3] Not available for intensive study.

4

The subgenera of avian malaria parasites

Four subgenera for the species of *Plasmodium* found in birds were established by Corradetti, Garnham and Laird (1963), whose original key ran:

1.	Round gametocytes	*Haemamoeba*
	Elongate gametocytes	2
2.	Schizogony in primitive blood-forming cells present	*Huffia*
	Schizogony in primitive blood-forming cells not present	3
3.	Large schizonts with plentiful cytoplasm	*Giovannolaia*
	Small schizonts with scanty cytoplasm	*Novyella*

Soon afterwards Garnham (1966) emended "not present" to "absent" in the above key and clarified point 3 by inserting "erythrocytic" before "schizonts" in both entries. While accepting that the scheme "may be as good as any that can be devised", Seed and Manwell (1977) further reworded the key by specifying the "relatively large asexual stages" of *Giovannolaia* by comparison with the "relatively small" ones of *Novyella*. They also asked, "Where, for example, does one draw the line between large and small asexual stages?" and "How does one allow for the fact that a given species may exhibit a somewhat different morphology in different host species?"

It is of course the nature of keys to invite such questions. The matter had been exhaustively discussed by Corradetti, Garnham and Laird (1963) while constructing this key and at the same time striving for brevity. At all events, Seed and Manwell (1977) agreed that "the groups listed as subgenera seem to be natural ones". They had already been accepted as such by other authors, including Greiner *et al.* (1975). However, Bennett, Whiteway and Woodworth-Lynas (1982) listed 75 published names for species and subspecies of avian plasmodia (recognizing 30 of these as valid and another as probably so) without reference to any subgenera at all.

Meanwhile, Sarker and Ray (1969; 1972) had described *Plasmodium coturnixae* from an Indian quail. In their second paper these authors described it as having elongate gametocytes and large schizonts, with

10–14 merozoites and scanty cytoplasm. Considering it "to occupy a place intermediate between *Novyella* and *Giovannolaia*", they designated their parasite as the type of a new subgenus, *Garnhamella*, and proposed modifying the Corradetti, Garnham and Laird (1963; Garnham emend. 1966) key as follows:

1.	Round gametocytes	*Haemamoeba*
	Elongate gametocytes	2
2.	Schizogony in primitive blood-forming cells present	*Huffia*
	Schizogony in primitive blood-forming cells absent	3
3.	Erythrocytic schizonts with plentiful cytoplasm and more than 14 merozoites	*Giovannolaia*
4.	Erythrocytic schizonts with scanty cytoplasm and less than 14 merozoites	*Garnhamella*
5.	Small erythrocytic schizonts with scanty cytoplasm and with 8 or fewer merozoites	*Novyella*

The problem with this proposal is two-fold. First, once ranges of merozoite number become specified criteria for subgeneric differentiation, the key loses flexibility. This risks unwarranted proliferation of subgenera, and indeed utter confusion. To illustrate the former, within the single subgenus *Haemamoeba*, the *Plasmodium relictum* complex and related species have merozoite numbers (individually variable with the strain) covering various portions of the spectrum between 6 and 32 (see Chapter 5 and Garnham 1966). As an example of utter confusion, the Sarkar and Ray key (note its points 3 and 4) has no place for members of *Giovannolaia* and the proposed subgenus *Garnhamella* with precisely 14 merozoites — a number commonly encounted among members of the former subgenus. Also, by specifying eight or fewer merozoites for *Novyella*, Sarkar and Ray (1972) automatically excluded one of the most important members of this subgenus, *P. nucleophilum*. In this the number quite often exceeds eight (p. 80). In Brazilian strains, it reaches 12 (p. 81). However, relevant taxonomic uncertainties will not arise. For Bennett, Whiteway and Woodworth-Lynas (1982) have already rejected "*P. coturnixae*" as ***incertae sedis***, and close study of the photomicrographs of Sarkar and Ray (1972) reveals that their proposed species may well have been described from a double infection. In this regard, Sarkar and Ray (1972) also mentioned discovering taxa resembling *P. (Haemamoeba) relictum* and *P. (Giovannolaia) circumflexum* in the same host in Calcutta. While they gave no details of either, their "*P. (G.) coturnixae*" combines features of *Haemamoeba* and *Giovannolaia*. It might also very possibly have been the same parasite that de Jong (1971) had well described as *P. (Novyella) dissanaikei* from Sri Lanka the year previously. The ***incertae sedis*** verdict of Bennett, Whiteway and Woodworth-Lynas (1982) must therefore stand, and *Garnhamella* must be rejected as a *nomen nudum*.

Despite the passage of more than three decades since Corradetti, Garnham and Laird (1963) proposed their allocation of the *Plasmodium* species of birds to four subgenera, the only plausible emendment since advanced leaves their classification still intact. It remains helpful in bringing a degree of order to the further study of a numerous (and otherwise disparate) assemblage of species. It is thus proposed to employ it in this book — but with two reservations. The first concerns *P. (Novyella) corradettii* n.sp., described in Chapter 7 and the second, *P. (N.) bertii* described by Gabaldon and Ulloa (1981). The latter, described from Venezuela (South American Realm, Region and Subregion), was overlooked by Bennett, Whiteway and Woodworth-Lynas (1982). Both exhibit features more characteristic of *Novyella* than any other of the four presently valid subgenera of avian plasmodia. At the same time, both display highly individual characteristics, and their distinctive gametocytes compare closely (p. 87). Following future life-history studies of *P. bertii* and *P. corradettii* n.sp., a fifth subgenus of bird malaria parasites could be called for. Meanwhile the Corradetti, Garnham and Laird classification is retained, but with a further emendment (to the third dichotomy) in the spirit of the suggestions of Seed and Manwell (1977), so that the key now reads:

1.	Round gametocytes	*Haemamoeba*
	Elongate gametocytes	2
2.	Schizogony in primitive blood-forming cells present	*Huffia*
	Schizogony in primitive blood-forming cells absent	3
3.	Erythrocytic schizonts usually larger than the host-cell nucleus, producing condensed merozoites of 1.0 μm or more in diameter, and seldom lacking conspicuous cytoplasm	*Giovannolaia*
	Erthrocytic schizonts usually smaller than the host-cell nucleus, producing condensed merozoites of less than 1.0 μm in diameter, and seldom having much cytoplasm	*Novyella*

5

Plasmodium (Haemamoeba)

Plasmodium (Haemamoeba) relictum (Grassi and Feletti 1891) *sensu lato*

The nominotypical subspecies of *P. relictum* (see next section in this chapter) is perhaps the most widespread and certainly the most mentioned of the avian malaria parasites. Many investigators have so identified virtually any bird *Plasmodium* with more-or-less round gametocytes causing radical displacement of the host-cell nucleus and some hypertrophy of the cell itself. Even in the absence of mature gametocytes, if much of the space within a similarly affected corpuscle is occupied by a large round to oval schizont staining largely reddish because its contents comprise many robust but often poorly differentiated nuclei, the same diagnosis is too often made.

Garnham (1966) stressed that in this variable species the number of merozoites differs from strain to strain. He cited various investigators for ranges from 8 to 12, 8 to 15, 16 to 24 and 14 to 32; and subsequently collaborated in a redescription of the nominotypical subspecies *P. relictum* by Corradetti *et al.* (1970).

This was based upon fresh material collected from the type host[1] and locality (Catania, Sicily). It confirmed the original data of Grassi and Feletti from four decades earlier; namely, that this species' schizonts form 10–24 merozoites, displace the host-cell nucleus and have pigment in black or dark brown granules which later assumes a golden glint. The photomicrographs of Corradetti *et al.* clearly illustrate the typical distortion and common rounding up of the parasitized red cell, and the latter's radically displaced nucleus — features also associated with other members of the subgenus *Haemamoeba.*

[1] *Passer hispaniolensis* (Temminck) 1820, the Spanish Sparrow [WN 2969] (in employing the scientific and popular names of Sibley and Monroe (1990) hereafter the terminal number within square brackets is preceded by "WN" as an abbreviation for "World List Number").

This raises uncertainty over the precise identification of "*P. relictum*" when variously described by earlier investigators dealing with Garnham's (1966) "strains" of this species in which mature schizonts (= segmenters) formed less than 10 or more than 24 merozoites. For example, Lawrence and Bearup (1961) reported *P. relictum* from fledglings of *Larus novaehollandiae* Stephens, Silver Gull [WN 8122.1] collected off Wollongong, New South Wales, Australia. Ensuing laboratory transmissions to (exotic) *Passer domesticus* and uninfected fledgling gulls led to what were represented as typical *P. relictum* infections. However, those of the former host had only 9–18 (av. 14.1) merozoites per segmenter, and those of the latter, 8–12 (av. 9.6). Importantly, it was also mentioned that in the field-collected bird with the highest parasitaemia the host-cell nucleus was occasionally expelled. Lawrence and Bearup ascribed the higher merozoite numbers from *Larus novaehollandiae* to their parasite's sojourn in an abnormal host. Laridae are certainly rare hosts to plasmodia (Bennett, Whiteway and Woodworth-Lynas 1982). The ranges and averages of merozoite numbers commonly differ from those of natural hosts, too, when *P. relictum* is transferred to laboratory canaries (Garnham 1966). It is in fact possible that Lawrence and Bearup were not dealing with the latter parasite at all but with *P. matutinum*, with which the data they provide appear more in accord. Garnham (1966) included this species with, for example, *P. cathemerium* and *P. subpraecox* among close relatives of *P. relictum* that "Even in recent years" had probably been confused with *P. relictum*.

Supporting Garnham's contention, Manwell, Allen and Kuntz (1976) refrained from making separate identifications of *P. relictum* and *P. cathemerium* from their Taiwan material. Instead, they simply lumped together 20 (25.6%) of their 78 *Plasmodium*-positive birds as *"cathemerium-relictum"*. It is unfortunate that the prime taxonomic character of *P. cathemerium*, the rod-like pigment granules, pointed at either end, of the sexual stages (especially the microgametocytes), is not always evident; so that if they "cannot be discerned, this would not necessarily mean that the parasite is not *P. cathemerium*" (Garnham 1966). Particularly as the latter parasite could only be (tentatively) identified from a single MAPS bird (not from Taiwan; see heading *"Plasmodium (Haemamoeba) cathemerium*" in this chapter), it is submitted that Manwell, Allen and Kuntz (1976) would have done better to allocate those 20 lumped-together infections as due to *P. relictum* **s.l.**

Fifteen (36.6%) of the 41 birds positive for *P. relictum* **s.l.** exhibited no other haematozoa. The 26 (63.4%) others had double or triple infections (Table 5.1). Nine (56.3%) of the 16 double infections, and nine (90%) of the 10 triple ones, included additional species of *Plasmodium*, two of which were associated in preparations from two different hosts (Table 5.1). *P. relictum* **s.l.** was accompanied by *P. vaughani* on eight occasions, by *P. rouxi* on five and by *P. nucleophilum* on four. *P. polare* occurred in two double infections, and *P. dissanaikei* in another. Of other haematozoan groups present in mixed infections with *P. relictum* **s.l.**, *Haemoproteus* occurred nine times. There were three findings of *Leucocytozoon*, two of microfilariae and one of *Trypanosoma*.

Table 5.1 Findings of *Plasmodium (Haemamoeba) relictum* ***sensu lato***

Host species[1]	Numbers recorded	Associated haematozoa[2]	Localities	Months
Argusianus argus	1	*H*	Gombak, Malaysia	January
Eudynamis scolopacea	1	*P.n.*	Palawan, Philippines	May
Ninox scutulata	1	*L*	Dalton Pass, Luzon, Philippines	October
Chalcophaps indica	1	mf	Palawan, Philippines	May
Chalcophaps indica	1	*P.v., P.n.*	Sara Buri, Thailand	January
Amaurornis phoenicurus	1	*P.d.*	Rantau Panjang, Malaysia	April
Amaurornis phoenicurus	1	*P.p.*	Rantau Panjang, Malaysia	April
Lanius cristatus	3	–	Ping-tung, Taiwan	September
Lanius cristatus	1	*H. lanii, P.v.*	Ping-tung, Taiwan	September
Lanius cristatus	1	–	Kabigan, Palawan, Philippines	October
Lanius cristatus	1	–	Aborlan, Palawan, Philippines	March
Lanius cristatus	2	–	Negros Oriental, Philippines	September
Lanius cristatus	1	–	Calatagan, Luzon, Philippines	September
Lanius cristatus	1	–	Laguna, Luzon, Philippines	October
Zoothera sibirica	1	*L*	Mt Brinchang, Malaysia	November
Zoothera sibirica	1	*P.v., P.r.*	Mt Brinchang, Malaysia	December
Copsychus niger	1	*H*, mf	Palawan, Philippines	May
Copsychus saularis	1	*P.v.*	Koh Kred, Pak Kred, Thailand	January
Copsychus saularis	1	*H*	Koh Kred, Pak Kred, Thailand	April
Luscinia cyane	1	*P.r.*	Subang, Malaysia	September
Luscinia cyane	1	–	Subang, Malaysia	November
Luscinia cyane	1	*P.v., P.r.*	Tsunoshima, Yamaguchi, Japan	May
Pycnonotus cafer	1	*L, P.v.*	Bharatpur, Rajasthan, India	October
Pycnonotus melanoleucos	1	*H, P.r.*	Sara Buri, Thailand	January
Prinia familiaris	1	–	Indonesia	March
Prinia flaviventris	1	*H. sylvae, P.r.*	Northern Thailand	January
Prinia hodgsonii	1	*H. sylvae*	Chiang Mai, Thailand	July
Acrocephalus aedon	1	*H*	Koh Kred, Pak Kred, Thailand	January
Acrocephalus aedon	1	*P.n.*	Chiang Mai, Thailand	January
Locustella lanceolata	1	*H, P.v.*	Pasi, Mindoro Oriental, Philippines	September
Trichastoma rostratum	1	–	Rantau Panjang, Malaysia	April
Trichastoma rostratum	1	*P.d.*	Rantau Panjang, Malaysia	March
Trichastoma rostratum	1	*P.p.*	Subang, Malaysia	August
Dicaeum cruentatum	1	*T, P.v.*	Kuala Kangsar, Malaysia	October
Ploceus philippinus	1	–	Nonthaburi, Thailand	August
Ploceus philippinus	1	*P.n.*	Kutch, India	March
Lonchura malacca	1	–	Camarines Norte, Luzon, Philippines	April
Emberiza elegans	1	–	Kwangyang, S. Korea	February
Totals 22 host species	41 individuals +ve *Plasmodium relictum* **s.l.**			

[1] Taxonomic order as in Table 2.2.

[2] *Trypanosoma (T), Haemoproteus (H,* with species name where possible), *Leucocytozoon (L), Plasmodium* [*P. polare (P.p.); P. dissanaikei (P.d.), P. vaughani (P.v.); P. rouxi (P.r.); P. nucleophilum (P.n.)*] and microfilariae (mf).

Thirty-four (82.9%) of the 41 infections were from passerines. Two of the remainder were from rails, two from doves, and one each from a typical owl, an Old World cuckoo and a pheasant. For the pheasant (a Great Argus) there are records of "*Plasmodium praecox*" (= *P. relictum* **s.l.**) (Scott 1928; Hamerton 1929) and *Plasmodium* sp. (Hamerton 1934). These antedate the description of *P. gallinaceum* (p. 38) which has been experimentally transmitted to pheasants (see Garnham 1966). Schizonts and gametocytes of *P. gallinaceum*, in a light infection such as the present one, are virtually inseparable in a thin blood smear from those of *P. relictum* **s.l.**

Most of the collecting stations featured in Table 5.1 are from the Philippines, Thailand and adjacent parts of Malaysia. In all of these the rainy season extends from June through October, while in only partly tropical Taiwan, the wettest months are June to August. These are also the times of peak mosquito populations, including avian malaria vectors — whatever these may eventually prove to be for each of the areas and avian hosts in question. The MAPS *Plasmodium* data are inadequate for meaningful evaluation of many of the issues involved, for example, the significance of altitudinal migration of resident birds in the further dispersal of haematozoa carried by long-distance migrants using the great Flyways. In this connection a pioneer study by Bauer (1939; 1941) conducted in the republic of Georgia in 1935–36 revealed that passerines wintering in valleys at about 400–500 m already harboured "*P. praecox*" (= *P. relictum* **s.l.**) by their spring movement to highland (about 1500–2500 m) breeding grounds. However, the lack of larval mosquito habitats in the dry uplands precluded transmission there. While *Plasmodium* sp? and *P. relictum* **s.l.** were recorded from MAPS slides made in all 12 months (Tables 3.1 and 5.1), the 41 Asian Tropical Subregion infections with the latter peaked at 22% of the annual total in September, when southward migration was reaching its height (McClure 1974; p. 49).

Plasmodium (Haemamoeba) relictum (Grassi and Feletti 1891) emend. Corradetti *et al.* 1970, nominotypical ssp. *relictum*

Under the *International Code of Zoological Nomenclature*, Third Edition (1985), Article 16 states that: "A scientific name proposed expressly as the name of a 'variety' or 'form' after 1960 is infrasubspecific and excluded from zoological nomenclature [Art. 1b (5)]; such proposal before 1961 does not prevent availability [Art. 45g]." Article 45 (g) (ii) indicates that such names published before 1961 are now ranked as subspecific. Their original rank is deemed to be such under Article 45 (f) (ii), which together with Article 45 (g) (ii) fully justifies the recognition of pre-1961 "varieties" of *P. relictum* as subspecies under the 1985 Code, although the present status of all but one of these ssp. *capistranoae* (Russell 1932; emend. Garnham 1966) is in contention. Under Article 47 (a) of the 1985 Code, a nominotypical subspecies therefore exists, containing the name-bearing type of the species, with the same author and date [Art. 46a], i.e., *P. relictum* (Grassi and Feletti 1891) ssp. *relictum* (Grassi and Feletti 1891). No type material having been preserved from the original Sicilian material from *Passer hispaniolensis*, (Corradetti *et al.* 1970) on redescribing *P. relictum*, deposited neotypes at the Wellcome Historical Museum of Medical Science, London, UK. Now properly termed "neohapantotypes" under the 1985 Code, these preparations (fully described on p. 124 of Garnham and Duggan 1986) are the responsibility of the Natural History Museum, London, UK, where they comprise part of the Garnham Collection of Malaria Parasites and Other Haemosporidia. They are of course neohapantotypes for the nominotypical subspecies *relictum* as well.

In the ten MAPS birds of nine species where the identification of ssp. *relictum* was felt justified (Table 5.2), both mature and immature red cells had been invaded (Corradetti *et al.* 1970). These corpuscles were variously distorted, and their nuclei were radically displaced and tilted (Figure 5.1). An erythroblast of *Otus lempiji* containing a small polar schizont in which nuclear division had only just begun was recorded as having its own nucleus displaced almost to the opposite pole. Garnham (1966) emphasized that dislodgement of the host-cell nucleus always occurs. However, he believed that "because there is a great variation in strains", merozoite number is an unreliable criterion for *P. relictum* "though the number will not be below eight and may be as high as thirty-two". Nevertheless, the subsequent (Corradetti *et al.* 1970) redescription of this species, to which he was party, specifies 10–24 (av. 14.1) merozoites per schizont, 10, 12, 14 and 16 being the commonest numbers. With only two exceptions the preparations listed in Table 5.2 conformed to the redescription of the schizonts, and also to that of the gametocytes, with their usually spherical or subspherical shape and round, black pigment granules.

One of the exceptions mentioned above concerned a single mature schizont exhibiting 32 merozoites, from an example of *Ninox philippensis*; the merozoite number of which was otherwise within the usual

Table 5.2 Findings of ***Plasmodium (Haemamoeba) relictum*** spp. ***relictum***

Host species[1] (individual positive records)	Associated haematozoa[2]	Localities	Months
Gallus gallus	*H., P.n., Ae*	Puerto Princessa, Palawan, Philippines	May
Ninox philippensis	*H. noctuae, P.f.*	Negros, Philippines	November
Otus lempiji	*P.f.*	Nakhon Ratchasima, Thailand	September
Pericrocotus divaricatus	–	Rantau Panjang, Malaysia	December
Dicrurus hottentottus	–	Central Thailand	November
Dicrurus hottentottus	*H, P.v., P.r.*	Central Thailand	January
Copsychus niger	*H. fallisi*, mf	Panagturan Point, Palawan, Philippines	May
Aplonis panayensis	*Ae, L, P.n.*, mf	Puerto Princessa, Palawan, Philippines	May
Pycnonotus blanfordi	*H*	Bang Phra, Cholburi, Thailand	June
Ploceus philippinus	*Ae, H. quelea*	Bang Phra, Cholburi, Thailand	June
Totals 9 host species	10 individuals +ve *P. relictum* ssp. *relictum*		

[1] Taxonomic order as in Table 2.2

[2] *Aegyptianella (Ae); Haemoproteus (H*, with species name where possible), *Leucocytozoon (L), Plasmodium* [*P. fallax (P.f.); P. vaughani (P.v.); P. rouxi (P.r.); P. nucleophilum (P.n.)*] and microfilariae (mf).

range of 10–14. This is inclined to be considered an aberrancy perhaps associated with the particular strain in an owl. The other exception concerns *Otus lempiji* with small schizonts having only eight chromatin masses present. These schizonts, although bearing a superficial resemblance to mature ones of *P. subpraecox* (p. 35) were actually only in mid-development and destined for a final chromatin division initiating the formation of 16 merozoites. The ssp. *relictum* gametocytes in this infection were also as described by Corradetti *et al.* (1970). The fact that only ten unqualified identifications of the latter subspecies could be made from the MAPS material in sharp contrast to 41 of *P. relictum* **s.l.** further reinforces Garnham's (1966) point about the very real difficulty of distinguishing the species (let alone the subspecies!) of *Haemamoeba* from one another, from blood smears alone.

In all, *P. (Giovannolaia) fallax, P. (Novyella) vaughani, P. (N.) rouxi* and *P. (N.) nucleophilum* were found variously associated with *P. relictum* ssp. *relictum*. There was no significant difficulty in distinguishing *P. relictum* from any of the four other members of its genus, nor from the five haemoproteids also encountered. *Haemoproteus noctuae* Celli and Sanfelice (emend. Bishop and Bennett 1989) is a frequent parasite of typical owls. It has already been recorded from the present host by Bishop and Bennett, who designated a *Ninox philippensis* blood film from Negros as a neohapantotype. They also recorded the second haemoproteid of the Strigidae, *H. syrnii* (Mayer; emend. Bishop and Bennett 1989) from the same host. *Haemoproteus fallisi* (Bennett and Campbell 1972) was reported from numerous other MAPS hosts including three other species of *Copsychus* in the original description. The description of *H. quelea* (Marullaz) has been emended by Bennett and Peirce (1991). Table 5.2 lists two quadruple haematozoan infections, a quintuple example being noteworthy.

Plasmodium (Haemamoeba) relictum **(Grassi and Feletti 1891) ssp.** ***capistranoae*** **Russell (1932) emend. Garnham (1966)**

Russell (1932b) described *P. capistrani* — which as he named it after his chief microscopist, Miss Ampara Capistrano, necessitated emendment to "*capistranoae*" as duly done by Garnham (1966) — at a time when there were only six well-recognized avian malaria parasites that have survived until now: *P. relictum, P. vaughani, P. cathemerium, P. rouxi, P. elongatum* and *P. circumflexum*. Important points that he made for the distinctiveness of his new taxon were that (i) both micro- and macrogametocytes are spherical, usually lying in the apex of the cell which is often distorted; (ii) the nucleus of the red cell is always pushed aside and may lie transversely or it may be absent; and (iii) pigment is abundant in gametocytes of both sexes, being scattered throughout the cytoplasm and seeming "to be more prominent than in the other species of malaria plasmodia"; while vacuoles are "not uncommon" in the developing stages, and segmenters, which are plentiful in the peripheral blood, form 8–16 merozoites. His type host was "*Excalfactoria lineata*", the "island painted quail". This is now recognized as *Coturnix [chinensis] chinensis* (Table 2.2), the Blue-breasted Quail [WN 3061]. The type locality was Novaliches (14.44N × 121.03E), somewhat north of Quezon City and northeast of Manila, Luzon, Philippines.

Obviously, the closest comparison was with *P. relictum*. The most important affinity with the closely related *P. cathemerium* was the presence (together with cone-shaped and spherical ones) of cylindrical pigment granules (see Laird and van Riper 1981, figure 17); which, however, were of only sporadic occurrence, and never actually spindle-shaped. A further point of resemblance between *P. cathemerium* and "*P. capistranoae*" was that both cause ejection of the host-cell nucleus far more frequently than does the nominotypical subspecies of *P. relictum*.

Several additional species of avian malaria parasites had been described by the time of publication of the first (and to date, only) book devoted to the subject. Those still surviving that were included in Hewitt's (1940) key to species identification, significantly "Based chiefly on the morphology in the vertebrate host, as seen in stained blood smears", are: *P. gallinaceum, P. fallax, P. nucleophilum, P. polare* and *P. lophurae*. Hewitt synonymized "*P. capistrani*" with *P. relictum*, but without "justifying" his opinion. Garnham (1966) presented cogent reasons why Russell's (1932b) parasite should be recognized as a valid subspecies of *P. relictum*, exhibiting as it does "certain morphological differences (e.g. ragged or polar gametocytes), a long sporogonic cycle, and incomplete cross immunity with the type" (i.e. the nominotypical subspecies). Laird and van Riper (1981) published additional information on *P. relictum* ssp. *capistranoae* from Hawaii, USA, which the organism may have entered accidentally in consequence of the introduction of *Coturnix chinensis* "from the Orient to Kauai in 1910" (Berger 1972). Bennett, Whiteway and Woodworth-Lynas (1982) accepted Garnham's (1966) opinion on the subspecific status of Russell's "species"; which at this time remains the only acceptable subspecies of *P. relictum* other than the nominotypical one.

Two examples of *Coturnix chinensis* sampled at Dalton Pass, north-central Luzon, Philippines, on 1 February 1965 proved positive for *P. relictum* ssp. *capistranoae*. Dalton Pass (about 1070 m) is on a major migration route for birds entering the Philippines from the north. MAPS ascertained that there are periodic movements of endemic tropical species over the mountains there, between Luzon's Central Plain and the northerly Cagayan Plain, netting 164 species during a 7 year study. Sixty were widespread tropical taxa, 57 Palaearctic migrants and 47 endemic species (McClure 1974). One of the Blue-breasted Quails (the type host of ssp. *capistranoae*, of which the type locality is some 180 km south of Dalton Pass) had an extremely low parasitaemia. The first mature segmenter was found after a 3.5 h oil-immersion search. Parasitaemia was quite heavy in the other bird, parasitized red cells averaging one per five oil-immersion fields (×15 oculars). Mature segmenters were common, gametocytes less so. In both cases there was an accompanying low-level infection of *Haemoproteus lophortyx* O'Roke, recently redescribed by Bennett and Peirce (1989), who designated a neohapantotype from a *Coturnix chinensis* netted at Dalton Pass during MAPS on 27 January 1968.

As described by Russell (1932b), signet-ring trophozoites are present in both erythroblasts and erythrocytes. They are usually located towards one pole of the host cell. With growth "vacuoles are not uncommon" as stated by Russell (Figures 5.2 and 5.3). Russell gave 8–16 as the merozoite number; Laird and van Riper (1981) found 6–16 in Hawaii. In the present instance it was 6–18. A count of 50 consecutive segmenters gave: 6 merozoites (2%); 8 merozoites (12%); 10 merozoites (26%); 12 merozoites (30%); 14 merozoites (20%); 16 merozoites (8%); and 18 merozoites (2%).

A feature of *P. relictum* spp. *capistranoae* not mentioned in the original description but evident in the present material is that tilting of the nucleus of the host red cell through an arc of 45° or more commonly occurs at the late trophozoite/early schizont stage.

Plasmodium (Haemamoeba) relictum (Grassi and Feletti 1891) subspecies *capistranoae* Russell emend. Garnham (1966) is formally redescribed as follows:

Type locality: Novaliches (14.44N × 121.03E), Luzon, Philippines.

Type host: (*Excalfactoria lineata*) = *Coturnix [chinensis] chinensis* (Linnaeus) 1766, Blue-breasted Quail [WN 3061].

Stages in peripheral blood: Trophozoites usually polar in erythroblasts or erythrocytes, occasionally two and rarely three in the same red cell of the type host, but up to eight in erythroblasts of recently infected, non-immune hosts. Host-cell distortion and radical nuclear displacement characteristic from late trophozoite/early schizont stage, when the red-cell nucleus is commonly tilted through some 45°. Prominent vacuoles quite common from early in schizont development onwards. Towards maturity the black pigment granules tending to clump roughly centrally. Segmenters with (rarely) six to (rarely) 18 merozoites, commonly 10 to 14. Gametocytes round or oval, with pigment generally scattered throughout the cytoplasm. Enucleation of the host corpuscle is frequent, being stimulated by both schizonts and gametocytes.

Periodicity: Not clearly defined, according to Russell (1932b).

Neohapantotype: Russell's type material of this subspecies not being known to have survived, a neohapantotype of *P. relictum* ssp. *capistranoae* is now designated. This slide already bears IRCAH No. 11050, and exhibits the heavier of the two infections derived from *Coturnix chinensis* at Dalton Pass, Luzon, on 1 February 1965.

Plasmodium (Haemamoeba) subpraecox Grassi and Feletti 1891 (?)

This organism has only been reported from a few species of Strigidae of Europe, the USA and North Africa. The hosts are listed by Bennett,

Whiteway and Woodworth-Lynas (1982) from earlier references. Garnham (1966) suggested the likelihood that a *Plasmodium* from the widespread Barn Owl — *Tyto alba* (Scopoli) 1769 [WN 365] — on the Pacific Island of "San Spirito" (= Espiritu Santo, Vanuatu) belongs to this species. His view was based on a personal communication from Barclay Maghee, indicating that the parasite formed "fairly large schizonts and round gametocytes in the erythrocytes". These data cannot really justify an identification narrower than *Plasmodium (Haemamoeba)* sp?

Only one MAPS slide exhibited a few parasites morphologically close to *P. subpraecox*. It was from an example of *Otus lempiji*, netted at Nakhon Ratchasima, Thailand, in September 1967. A small schizont from it, with ten nuclei distributed peripherally and occasioning only slight host-cell nuclear displacement, is illustrated in Figure 5.4. This parasite much resembles that of Garnham's (1966) figure 14, plate XLIV, except for the latter's having caused 90° twisting and more marked displacement of the erythrocyte nucleus. However, Figure 5.4 actually shows a schizont of *P. (Giovannolaia) fallax* (also see Figures 6.1 and 6.2) very much like the one causing minimal displacement of the red cell nucleus, seen in Garnham's (1966) figure 14, plate LII. All blood stages of *P. fallax* abounded on the *O. lempiji* slide, which also bore *Haemoproteus noctuae* Celli and Sanfelice as redescribed by Bishop and Bennett (1989) — and a few typical gametocytes and (Figure 5.1) schizonts (forming 10–24 merozoites, average 16) of *P. relictum* ssp. *relictum*. The last-mentioned species caused its characteristic effects on host erythrocytes, agreeing in all respects with its redescription by Corradetti *et al.* (1970).

The triple infection under discussion (see Table 5.2, second entry) well illustrates the difficulties involved in determining the identities of avian malaria parasites when more than one species is present. Besides the possibility of confusion between *P. subpraecox* and *P. fallax* illustrated in Figure 5.4, three schizonts and a macrogametocyte of *P. relictum* ssp. *relictum* at the lower end of this species' size range might equally well have been listed as the first-mentioned species in the absence of other plasmodia! A major factor influencing Garnham's (1966) contention that *P. subpraecox* merits separate species status within subgenus *Haemamoeba* was that it "appears to be confined to the owl, and this bird is practically insusceptible to the passerine *P. relictum*". The present example does not support this statement. Neither do the MAPS occurrences of *P. relictum* **s.l.** in the Brown Hawk-Owl (*Ninox scutulata*) listed in Table 5.1 and of ssp. *relictum* in the Philippine Hawk-Owl (*N. philippensis*) of Table 5.2. Furthermore, *P. relictum* **s.l.** is far from being restricted to passerines, as witness such MAPS records as those of Table 5.1 from *Argusianus argus* (Phasianidae), *Eudynamis scolopacea* (Cuculidae), *Chalcophaps indica* (Columbidae) and *Amaurornis phoenicurus* (Rallidae).

The presence of a few *subpraecox*-like parasites in the multiple haematozoan infection discussed earlier from *Otus lempiji* is clearly insufficient evidence to justify a record of this organism from Thailand. *P. subpraecox* thus remains unknown from the Asian Tropical Subregion. The incident illustrates the care that must always be taken in allocating names to avian malaria parasites studied only in field-collected blood films. Suggesting as it does the virtual impossibility of distinguishing *P. subpraecox* from *P. relictum* and even small schizonts of *P. fallax* in mixed infections in such blood films, one must doubt the desirability of separate species rank for *P. subpraecox*.

Especially as "when *P. subpraecox* is inoculated into canaries, it becomes indistinguishable from *P. relictum*" (Garnham 1966), it seems more realistic at this time to identify plasmodia with its morphological characteristics as *P. relictum* **s.l.**

Plasmodium (Haemamoeba) cathemerium Hartman 1927 (?)

As seen in smears of peripheral blood, *P. cathemerium* much resembles *P. relictum* **s.l.** Signet-ring trophozoites seldom occur in either, and in normal hosts the younger stages are solid looking little bodies (usually within young erythrocytes), often more or less polar in location. Developing schizonts of both may show relatively slight vacuolation. From 8 to 24 merozoites develop in the large schizonts of *P. cathemerium* according to Garnham (1966); Hewitt (1940) gives 6–24. These figures are similar to those of *P. relictum* **s.l.**, and in both organisms the average merozoite number is commonly 14 or 16. The round to oval mature gametocytes are also much the same in both cases, with the important difference that in *P. cathemerium* the pigment granules of gametocytes (particularly the microgametocytes, according to Garnham's 1966 analysis of the available data) are usually in the form of elongate spindles. Where they occur, these are immediately distinguishable from the round granules of *P. relictum* and its subspecies. Schizonts and gametocytes of the latter taxa and *P. cathemerium* both cause radical displacement and/or tilting of the host-cell nucleus, together with alteration of the outline of the erythrocyte itself. Expulsion of the host-cell nucleus occurs commonly, as in *P. relictum* **s.l.** and *P. matutinum*.

The outstanding morphological grounds for the recognition of *P. cathemerium* in Giemsa-stained blood films are two-fold. First, the presence of elongate, spindle-shaped granules of deep brown pigment in the sexual stages, particularly the microgametocytes (p. 37), and second, 24 h periodicity characterized by late-evening segmentation (Taliaferro 1925) in contrast to the asynchronous schizogonic cycle in the blood of *P. relictum* **s.l.** As for a variety of reasons tropical field collections of avian blood smears have generally been made in daylight, those of MAPS being no exception, the resultant slides have not, therefore, yielded the necessary periodicity data to help pinpoint *P. cathemerium*. The distinctive (although according to Garnham 1966, not always evident) shape of the pigment granules of *P. cathemerium* has thus remained the key character for recognition of this species.

One MAPS bird only, an example of *Lonchura malacca* netted on 27 April 1965 in Camarines Norte, Luzon, Philippines, harboured what was possibly a chronic infection with *P. cathemerium*. No other haematozoa were present, and just four parasites, three of them quite early microgametocytes (Figure 5.5) were discovered in almost 4 h of searching the entire smear. They and a macrogametocyte all exhibited elongate and sometimes terminally tapered pigment granules of brownish-black colour. An example of *Copsychus saularis* from Subang, Malaysia (25 June 1962) had a quadruple infection (Table 7.1) of *Haemoproteus fallisi* Bennett and Campbell (1972), *Plasmodium vaughani, P. rouxi* and a single example of *P. (Haemamoeba)* sp. The latter was a round microgametocyte which had appreciably displaced and tilted the red-cell nucleus, and its brownish-black pigment granules were rod-like. The third slide was from a Baya Weaver, *Ploceus philippinus*, from Bang Phra, Cholburi, Thailand (23 June 1967). It yielded a triple infection of *P. relictum* spp. *relictum, Haemoproteus quelea* (p. 32) and *Aegyptianella* sp. (Table 5.2). The first-mentioned was common. It was represented by trophozoites, schizonts, and separated merozoites still confined within the erythrocyte membrane. In one of the latter cases only eight merozoites were present. Counts from 29 others gave a range of 10–24 (av. 12). Three elongate spindles of pigment were present in one maturing schizont only. Considered by itself the latter certainly brought *P. cathemerium* to mind, but no supporting evidence was found, and the range of life-history stages on the slide accorded with the asynchronicity of *P. relictum* ssp. *relictum*.

The evidence from the second and third of the above birds is considered too insubstantial for an identification of *P. cathemerium*. That from the first, though, despite the fact that the parasite was represented on the *Lonchura malacca* slide only by four gametocytes (which while slim evidence for synchronicity at least does not suggest asynchronicity), could perhaps be held to justify tentative determination of this avian malaria parasite. However, *P. relictum* **s.l.** seems wiser.

There is no record of *P. cathemerium* from a natural host in the Asian Tropical Subregion, but there is a published reference to its earlier presence in Luzon, the Philippines island where the present finding was made. In connection with Russell's (1932b) experimental studies of *P. relictum* ssp. *capistranoae* in Manila, he imported a strain of the former parasite descended from Hartman's (1927) original one from Baltimore, Maryland, and sent to him by Dr. Clay G. Huff. As nicely put by Garnham (1966) this strain remained "a favoured laboratory plaything" for some 20 years after its 1924 discovery. One must wonder, therefore, whether the Baltimore strain was maintained in Manila until the disruption of the January 1942 Japanese occupation of that city during World War II? And if so, whether some local vector such as *Culex quinquefasciatus* perhaps became infected from parasitized laboratory birds in the midst of chaos, subsequently transmitting *P. cathemerium* to free-living passerines (such as the abundant and peridomestic *L. malacca*) nearby? While the remote possibility seems worth mentioning, the author doubts whether it happened. For had it done so on a large island with the diverse avian *Plasmodium* fauna revealed by MAPS, surely much more evidence for the presence of a rather recently established species would have been forthcoming?

All that can be concluded from the very scanty data produced for *P. cathemerium* by MAPS is that this species has at best a very spotty distribution in the Asian Tropical Subregion. This suggests occasional accidental establishments, especially via migratory birds that had become parasitized while nesting somewhere in Eurasia, from which there are numerous records (see Garnham 1966) and particularly more recent western-central Asian findings. These include those of Zeiniev (1975a;b) from Azerbaydzhan, and from Central Asia, those of Subkhonov (1972a;b) from Tadzhikistan, and Yakunin (1976) and Yakunin and Zhazyltaev (1977) from Kazakhstan. Those from Kazakhstan are especially thought provoking (always remembering the real difficulty of making certain identifications of *P. cathemerium* from field-collected blood smears alone) in that among them are reports of this passerine parasite from such novel hosts as nightjars, pigeons and doves.

At all events, none of the three species of birds discussed herein harbouring or appearing to harbour *P. cathemerium* in the Asian Tropical Subregion are migratory. Two of them (*Ploceus philippinus* and *Lonchura malacca*) have been found by leg banding to travel relatively short distances (up to some 200 km and 160 km, respectively) over many months. *Copsychus saularis* is "very sedentary" with local recaptures for up to 72 months (McClure 1974).

Plasmodium (Haemamoeba) gallinaceum Brumpt 1935 (?)

The type host of *P. gallinaceum* Brumpt (1935) is the Domestic Fowl, to which it is generally considered to be restricted. Most nowadays follow Delacour (1965) in regarding the Domestic Fowl as derived from *Gallus [gallus] gallus* (Linnaeus) 1758, the Red Junglefowl [WN 309.4]. The Red Junglefowl is the most widespread of the four wild taxa of *Gallus*, occurring today from northwestern India to southern China and Hainan, and to Sumatra and Java (Crawford 1984). Some still claim a polyphyletic origin for the domesticated bird, applying to it the widely abandoned name of *G. domesticus*, which Sibley and Monroe (1990) do not recognize. However, while hybrids have resulted from the mating of all four wild taxa with the Domestic Fowl (Gray 1958), only those from the latter and Red Junglefowl are fully viable and reproduce normally (Crawford 1984).

There is evidence that in former times the range of the Red Junglefowl was much wider than now. Thus Ho (1977) discusses recent discoveries of *G. gallus* bones giving a radiocarbon date of 4398 ± 100 BP, from Lan-chou, Kansu (36.01N × 103.45E, approaching Mongolia's southern border). Crawford (1984) considered it unclear whether these bones were from wild or domesticated *Gallus*. He concluded that if they were indeed from the latter and therefore evidence that "Chinese domestication of chickens was the first, presumably that stock did not persist or it remained isolated". That aside, Zeuner (1963) presented archaeological evidence from the early Bronze Age Harappá culture in support of his contention that full domestication had been achieved in the Indus Valley by about 4000 BP. The relevant material from Mohenjo-Daro (27.17N × 68.14E), Pakistan ranged from a clay figurine of a hen with a food dish, to *G. gallus* bones much larger than those of wild junglefowl. Two cocks in fighting stance on a seal from the same site may have been intended for either the Red Junglefowl or *Gallus [gallus] sonneratii*, the Grey Junglefowl [WN 3097] (refs in Zeuner 1963).

A period of no more than 4000–4500 years is thus the most that can be allowed for the evolution of *Plasmodium gallinaceum*, failing a natural reservoir. On the basis of their discovery of a *P. relictum*-like parasite in one of 40 examples of *Gallus sonneratii* in Madras, India, and its successful subinoculation into chicks, Shortt *et al.* (1941) believed that they had found the natural host of *P. gallinaceum*. From this single event, Garnham (1966) declared that "The natural host of *P. gallinaceum* is the junglefowl, different species of which occur in the enzootic regions of the East". Fernando and Dissanaike (1974; 1975) identified both *P. gallinaceum* and *P. juxtanucleare* from the Red Junglefowl in Pahang, Malaysia, describing a pleomorphic form of the former. Fernando and Dissanaike's (1975) figures 2e–j actually illustrate *P. (Giovannolaia) circumflexum*, present in mixed infection with a *Haemamoeba*. The latter, as their merozoite range for both taxa was given as 13–35, cannot have been *P. gallinaceum*, the usual merozoite number for which is 16–20 (Garnham 1966); Hewitt (1940) gave the range as 8–30. It is considered that the *Haemamoeba* reported from the Malaysian Red Junglefowl was probably *P. relictum* **s.l.**, but as the uppermost merozoite number for a strain of this species was given by Giovannola (1939) as 32, a safer determination would be simply *P. (Haemamoeba)* sp?

Its high pathogenicity to chicks of the Domestic Fowl is the only certain characteristic differentiating *P. gallinaceum* from *P. relictum* **s.l.** Despite Garnham's (1966) assertion that "The presence in the blood of a domestic hen of a large malaria parasite, with numerous merozoites, spherical gametocytes and causing displacement of the host cell nucleus is an almost certain indication of *P. gallinaceum*", that morphological description applies equally well to *P. relictum* **s.l.**

One of 17 MAPS Red Junglefowls was blood-smeared near Puerto Princessa, Palawan, Philippines, on 24 May 1962. It harboured a triple infection (Table 7.3) of which the other components were *P. nucleophilum* and *Aegyptianella* sp. An Asian Glossy Starling (*Aplonis panayensis*) sampled that day in the same area (Tables 5.2 and 7.3) had a quintuple infection of *P. nucleophilum*, *P. relictum* ssp. *relictum*, an *Aegyptianella* morphologically indistinguishable from *A. pullorum*, a *Leucocytozoon* and microfilariae. The *P. nucleophilum* of the Palawan Red Junglefowl will be considered in Chapter 7. Its *Haemamoeba*, seen in Figures 5.6–5.8, had the undermentioned characteristics.

Parasitaemia was light, indicating a chronic infection. Synchronicity was not well marked, as trophozoites, schizonts and gametocytes were present simultaneously. Initially, the trophozoites were solidly oval, always lacking the clear central zone of the signet-ring forms so characteristic of various other avian malaria parasites, particularly those of subgenus *Novyella*. The trophozoites were usually polar or lateral to the normally positioned nucleus of the host cell. As early schizonts became evident with a measure of vacuolation and the start of chromatin division, displacement and tilting of the erythrocyte nucleus occurred (Figure 5.6). With further development (Figures 5.7 and 5.8) 8, 12 or 14 chromatin masses differentiated before the final division, the parasitized corpuscles being variously distorted and showing marked nuclear displacement. The few segmenters seen were in process of forming 16, 24 or 30 merozoites. The 30 merozoite figure is high for *P. relictum* ssp. *relictum*, in which, however, as many as 32 sometimes occur (Garnham 1966) and in fact did so in a MAPS *Ninox philippensis* slide (p. 31). One point not in accord with the latter author's description of the asexual cycle of *P. gallinaceum* in the blood, is his reference to the nucleus of the host cell remaining unchanged in position when early schizonts with a single vacuole are at the stage seen in Figure 5.6. Gametocytes seen in the Puerto Princessa slide had a few round, black pigment granules, caused radical tilting of the host-cell nucleus, and displaced it to or near the erythrocyte membrane. Their shape was round, oval or sometimes decidedly indented through pressing against the displaced nucleus. These things are in agreement with published descriptions of both *P. gallinaceum* and *P. relictum* ssp. *relictum*, and are also characteristic of the infection of the latter in the Asian Glossy Starling sampled on the same day and at the same place.

The Red Junglefowl and Asian Glossy Starling are both birds of the forest edge and second growth, bordering on grasslands and farmlands (Sibley and Monroe 1990). It seems reasonable to suppose that the closely associated examples of each from Puerto Princessa had been exposed to the same species of vectors, notably the locally common *Aedes aegypti* and *Culex quinquefasciatus* (= *pipiens fatigans*) which are good vectors of the above two malaria parasites. Short of assuming simply from its occurrence in *Gallus gallus* that the *Haemamoeba* under discussion is ***ipso facto*** *P. gallinaceum*, it is submitted that the data presented herein combine to support a confident identification of *P. relictum* ssp. *relictum*.

It should be mentioned that there is disagreement over whether the Red Junglefowl is indigenous or exotic in the Philippines. The present consensus is expressed by Sibley and Monroe (1990) who concede a *possible* importation to these islands. While conceding that the bird may have been originally imported — this might have taken place about 3000 BP when peoples of Malaysian stock were beginning to displace the earlier Negrito population — Parkes (1962) believed it to be indigenous. His reasoning was that the Red Junglefowl is not only present throughout the Philippines archipelago but also is visibly differentiated from populations elsewhere.

No Domestic Fowls were included in the MAPS project, but plasmodia "in all likelihood" referable to *P. gallinaceum* were reported from 125 (11.9%) of 1047 Philippines examples by Africa *et al.* (1940). Records from elsewhere in the Asian Tropical Subregion involve Domestic Fowls from the type locality of this parasite, Nhatrang (Vietnam), through India, Sri Lanka, Malaysia (including Sabah, Borneo) to Indonesia. Garnham (1966) provides relevant references. He states that records of *P. gallinaceum* "outside Asia are few and of doubtful significance", and stresses that epidemics with high mortality due to the resultant disease in Domestic Fowls have only occurred when the latter have been imported to the endemic area from elsewhere. "Elsewhere" in this context obviously includes regions such as Europe and Africa where Domestic Fowls had become established (following their arrival from Asia) 2000 years ago (Zeuner 1963). Loss of immunity over such a period is a reasonable expectation, and it was wise of Adene and Dipeolu (1981) to identify a malaria parasite from this host at Ibadan, Nigeria, simply as *Plasmodium* sp. Theirs was the sole published finding of a malaria parasite from *Gallus gallus* in sub-saharan Africa to be discovered in a recent comprehensive survey of poultry parasites conducted by the Pathology Section, Onderstepoort Veterinary Institute (Huchzermeyer 1993). Earlier reports from North and West Africa were questioned by Garnham (1966), who also mentioned that the only American field reports of parasites resembling *P. gallinaceum* were probably due to the inadvertent release of laboratory-infected chickens.

To summarize, it can be argued that an Asian Tropical Subregion strain of *Plasmodium relictum* **s.l.** became differentiated in domesticating *Gallus gallus* 4–5 millennia ago. That differentiation, however, did not extend to recognition in our day of separate morphological characteristics in blood smears between *P. gallinaceum* and *P. relictum* **s.l.** Why, therefore, bearing in mind the close ecological overlap between these taxa and many peridomestic hosts of the latter, must a specific differentiation be maintained? The case of the Puerto Princessa coincidence of a Red Junglefowl and an Asian Glossy Starling bearing morphologically inseparable *P. (Haemamoeba)* malaria parasites has been stated in this section, and will be taken up again in Chapter 7 with regard to *P. nucleophilum* and *P. juxtanucleare.*

A second such case of ecological coincidence between the Domestic Fowl and a locally common associate had been noticed by Bisseru and Lim (1971). They claimed to have found both *P. gallinaceum* and the second Domestic Fowl malaria parasite, *P. (Novyella) juxtanucleare*, in a very prevalent associate of this bird in the Asian Tropical Subregion. The locality was Klang, Malaysia, and the peridomestic associate was *Corvus splendens*, the House Crow [WN 2449]. There is nothing in the paper of Bisseru and Lim (1971) to suggest that their *Haemamoeba* was anything other than *P. relictum* **s.l.**; which has often been reported from species of *Corvus* (Bennett, Whiteway and Woodworth–Lynas 1982) and which Nandi (1978) was soon to identify from Indian *C. splendens.* It is appropriate that Fernando and Dissanaike (1975) should have pointed to *C. splendens* as an example of erroneous identifications of *P. gallinaceum*; for as in the former, *P. relictum* **s.l.** is often found in association with *P. (Novyella)* and *Aegyptianella* (of a species morphologically inseparable from *A. pullorum*) in common wild birds that so often share the peridomestic environment of the Domestic Fowl in the Asian Tropical Subregion. The *Novyella* parasitizing these wild hosts is *P. (N.) nucleophilum*, the closest relative of *P. juxtanucleare* (see pp. 82–84).

Plasmodium (Haemamoeba) matutinum (Huff 1937) emend. Corradetti *et al.* 1960

Forty-three birds of sixteen host species were found to harbour *P. matutinum*, from India, Malaysia and Thailand to South Korea, Taiwan and the Philippines (Table 5.3). This species was thus a close contender with *P. relictum* **s.l.** (from 41 birds of 22 host species ranging from India, Malaysia, Thailand and Indonesia to Japan, South Korea, Taiwan and the Philippines; Table 5.1) for the role of commonest, most host-tolerant and widest ranging of the *Haemamoeba* present in the MAPS collections. Uegaki's (1930) illustrations suggest that he might have encountered *P. matutinum* in Malaysian Passeridae. Of the 43 Asian Tropical Subregion birds with *P. matutinum* (Table 5.3), 28% were sampled during the period of southward migration for wintering (September–November), mostly (23%) in September alone.

Table 5.3 Findings of ***Plasmodium (Haemamoeba) matutinum***

Host species[1] (individual positive records)	Associated haematozoa[2]	Localities	Months
Chalcophaps indica	*T, P.n.*	Tarabanan, Palawan, Philippines	May
Treron curvirostra	*P.v.*	Kuala Lumpur, Malaysia (captive)	December
Lanius cristatus	–	Sibulan, Negros Oriental, Philippines	September
Lanius cristatus	–	Sibulan, Negros Oriental, Philippines	September
Lanius cristatus	–	Sibulan, Negros Oriental, Philippines	September
Lanius cristatus	–	Camp Lookout, Negros Oriental, Philippines	September
Lanius cristatus	–	Siaton, Negros Oriental, Philippines	February
Lanius cristatus	*H. lanii, P.v.*	Siaton, Negros Oriental, Philippines	January
Lanius cristatus	*H. lanii*	Palawan, Philippines	May
Lanius cristatus	–	Aborlan, Palawan, Philippines	?
Lanius cristatus	*P.r.*	Aborlan, Palawan, Philippines	August
Lanius cristatus	*H. lanii*	Aborlan, Palawan, Philippines	April
Lanius cristatus	*H. lanii*	Batangas, Luzon, Philippines	April
Lanius cristatus	*H. lanii*	Batangas, Luzon, Philippines	April
Lanius cristatus	*H. lanii, P.v.*	Calatagan, Luzon, Philippines	September
Lanius cristatus	–	Ping-tung, Taiwan	September
Lanius cristatus	*H. lanii, P.p.*	Subang, Malaysia	September
Lanius cristatus	*P.p.*	Subang, Malaysia	?
Lanius cristatus	*H. lanii*	Chiang Mai, Thailand	January
Lanius schach ¶ nasutus	–	Dalton Pass, Luzon, Philippines	June
Lanius validirostris	*H. lanii*	Mindoro, Philippines	September
Lanius validirostris	*H. lanii*	Mindoro, Philippines	September
Copsychus saularis	–	Mahabaleshwar, India	March
Copsychus saularis	*P.r.*	Rantau Panjang, Malaysia	January
Copsychus saularis	*P.r., P.v.*	Rantau Panjang, Malaysia	January
Copsychus saularis	–	Rantau Panjang, Malaysia	April
Copsychus saularis	*P.r.*	Rantau Panjang, Malaysia	May
Copsychus saularis	*P.r.*	Rantau Panjang, Malaysia	September
Luscinia cyane	*P.r., At*	Subang, Malaysia	November

Table 5.3 *(cont.)*

Host species[1] (individual positive records)	Associated haematozoa[2]	Localities	Months
Pycnonotus simplex	*H. octocompsae* *P.ci.*	Subang, Malaysia	July
Zosterops japonicus	*P.n., P.v.*	Chiang Mai, Thailand	December
Trichastoma rostratum	*P.d., P.e., At*	Rantau Panjang, Malaysia	March
Nectarinia jugularis	–	Northern Thailand	August
Nectarinia jugularis	*P.p.*	Tarabanan, Palawan, Philippines	May
Nectarinia jugularis	*P.n., P.co.*	Tarabanan, Palawan, Philippines	May
Nectarinia jugularis	*P.v.*	Puerto Princessa, Palawan, Philippines	May
Motacilla alba	*P.d.*	Rajasthan, India	January
Ploceus manyar	*P.n.*	Bangkok, Thailand	March
Ploceus philippinus	–	Chiang Mai, Thailand	December
Ploceus philippinus	*H. quelea, L.*	Chiang Mai, Thailand	December
Ploceus philippinus	*H. quelea*	Bang Phra, Cholburi, Thailand	September
Ploceus philippinus	*H. quelea, P.n.*	Bang Phra, Cholburi, Thailand	August
Lonchura malacca	–	Subang, Malaysia	November
Emberiza fucata	–	Chinchup-Myun, S. Korea	July
Totals 16 host species	43 individuals +ve *P. matutinum*		

[1] Taxonomic order as in Table 2.2.

[2] *Trypanosoma (T), Haemoproteus* (*H*, with species name), *Leucocytozoon (L), Plasmodium* [*P. circumflexum (P.ci.); P. polare (P.p.); P. dissanaikei (P.d.); P. vaughani (P.v.); P. rouxi (P.r.); P. nucleophilum (P.n.); P. corradettii* n.sp. *(P.co.), P. elongatum (P.e.)*] and *Atoxoplasma (At).*

Originally isolated in Kansas, Illinois, USA, from a thrush (then Turdidae, now Muscicapidae), the American Robin, *Turdus migratorius migratorius* Linnaeus 1766 [WN 761], this parasite was described as a subspecies of *P. relictum* by Huff (1937). It was soon found to be widely distributed in the United States, where it was the subject of much laboratory research in the heyday of avian malariology. In this period it was found in two other native thrushes and *Passer domesticus* in the United States, and in two Mexican birds, a finch and a pigeon (Garnham 1966). With further respect to the Columbiformes, as reports of avian malaria from pigeons and doves had continued to mount, all but two had been ascribed to *P. matutinum* according to the interpretation by Garnham (1966) of Levine's (1962) geographical review of the haematozoa of this avian order. By 1962, Corradetti, Neri and Scanga (1960) had published a redescription of Huff's (1937) parasite, elevating it to the status of a full species. Their redescription was overlooked by Levine (1962), who continued to refer almost all columbiform *Plasmodium* findings to *P. relictum*.

The Corradetti, Neri and Scanga (1960) redescription was based on an original finding from another thrush, captured in Tuscany. This was *Turdus iliacus* Linnaeus 1766, the Redwing [WN 760], the above redescription of *P. matutinum* from which follows.

The known strains of *P. matutinum* exhibit a 24 h cycle on subinoculation to laboratory canaries. They thereby differ from *P. relictum* **s.l.** with its asynchronous cycle of 30–36 h, and from *P. gallinaceum* with its fairly synchronous 36 h cycle. However, their 24 h periodicity is shared by *P. subpraecox, P. cathemerium* and *P. giovannolai* (figures from summaries of data in Garnham 1966). Like the last three species and also *P. relictum* ssp. *capistranoae* and *P. gallinaceum, P. matutinum* commonly exhibits multiple invasion of the host erythrocyte, which may be either mature or immature; as in Figure 5.9, in which a newly invaded merozoite is seen to the right of the cell. Table 5.3 lists the 43 birds of 16 host species harbouring *P. matutinum* in the MAPS collections.

Early trophozoites (Figure 5.9 left-hand example) are solid, oval bodies with abundant cytoplasm. Three were seen, all located towards the poles of one host cell (an erythroblast), in a preparation from *Lanius cristatus* secured at Subang, Malaysia, on 21 September 1962. Double invasions were quite common in other hosts. A conspicuous vacuole appears with further growth, the parasite's outline becoming irregular and its chromatin conspicuous (Figure 5.10). By this stage, displacement of the nucleus of the host cell and the latter's hypertrophy are marked. The nucleus is often tilted through 30°–45° (Figures 5.11 and 5.14). In the former figure, division of the parasite's chromatin has begun, and vacuolation of its cytoplasm has become more prominent. Figure 5.12 illustrates (in this instance small) the "punched-out" vacuoles of a larger schizont. The arrow of Figure 5.13 points to such a vacuole in a schizont with chromatin division into four in progress, within an immature red cell. Eight chromatin masses are evident in the schizonts of Figures 5.14 and 5.15, and 14 in that of Figure 5.16. Figures 5.15 and 5.16 also show how maturing schizonts cram the displaced nucleus against the host-cell membrane.

Figure 5.17 illustrates a 12-merozoite segmenter. An accurate count is scarcely possible from the photomicrograph, as some of the merozoites, which have not yet begun to condense, obscure others. In Figure 5.18, the (14) dispersed merozoites have condensed to their final spherical shape (compare the newly invaded one of Figure 5.9). Also in the previous example, schizogony has been completed in a polychromatophil erythroblast. The fine granules of blackish pigment of *P. matutinum* are often inconspicuous in trophozoites and the younger schizonts. As the latter mature, though, pigment clumps into a conspicuous mass which is often central or nearly so within the peripherally arranged merozoites (Figure 5.19), but sometimes appreciably (Figure 5.20) or markedly (Figure 5.21) eccentric. From 8 to 18 merozoites are formed by segmentation, the most characteristic numbers being 14 and 16. As many as 18 merozoites were seen once only. This was in a *Lanius validirostris* slide from Mindoro, Philippines. At the other end of the scale a number just below the usual *P. matutinum* range of 10–22 (Garnham 1966) was less rare. Thus mature schizonts and segmenters exhibiting only eight merozoites were seen in four passerine hosts and seven individual birds. These were: three *Lanius cristatus*, from two major islands of the Philippines, Negros Oriental (Siaton, 16 January 1965; Sibulan, 25 September 1961) and Palawan

(Aborlan, 13 May 1962); two *Nectarinia jugularis*, both from Palawan (Puerto Princessa, 24 May 1962; Tarabanan, 13 May 1962); a *Motacilla alba* from Rajasthan, India (9 January 1968) and a *Ploceus philippinus* from Bang Phra, Cholburi, Thailand (1 September 1966).

Otherwise, the schizonts found fell within the usual *P. matutinum* range, having 10–18 merozoites with 14 or 16 being the numbers most commonly encountered. A typical spread from 50 counted in the heaviest infection in *Lanius cristatus* was eight merozoites (three examples, or 6%); 10 (six, or 12%); 12 (10, or 20%); 14 (14, or 28%); and 16 (17, or 34%). The abrupt fall-off following 16 is puzzling, suggesting as it does that there should be a declining incidence in numbers from there to something closer to the usual *P. matutinum* upper limit of 22.

In a number of infections, developing schizonts with eight large and diffuse chromatin masses were present. These were clearly destined for a further division, and the initiation of 16 merozoites. So care was taken in investigating the minimum numbers of merozoites in mature schizonts, to accept as counts of eight only examples on the brink of segmentation; or else scattering, condensed merozoites following segmentation (like the 14-merozoite example of Figure 5.18).

One of the schizonts on the brink of segmentation, in the slide from *Motacilla alba* from Rajasthan (probably from accompanying notes, Bharatpur, 27.14N × 77.28E) had only eight as yet uncondensed merozoites. It was unusually small, not in fact much larger than one of its host's erythrocyte nuclei. But despite its diminutive size, its presence had resulted in the enucleation of the host red cell. Nuclear expulsion had been as effectively achieved in erythrocytes of *Lanius cristatus, Luscinia cyane* and *Zosterops japonicus*, now empty except for much larger, 16-nucleate segmenters. All these were in every way characteristic of *P. matutinum*, down to the single clump of pigment, blackish or greenish-black, located centrally to almost peripherally as already described. Just prior to segmentation the cell membrane of an enucleated erythrocyte sometimes loses its shape, presumably through parasite-induced fragility (Figure 5.22).

Immature gametocytes of *P. matutinum*, like the younger schizonts with which it is easy to confuse them (Wolfson 1937), cause radical displacement and tilting of the host-cell nucleus. Initially often of highly irregular outline and exhibiting mostly peripheral pigment granules (Figure 5.23), they soon become more or less oval (Figure 5.24) prior to rounding up at maturity (Figures 5.25–5.27), by which stage the parasitized erythrocyte has usually lost its nucleus (Figure 5.26).

In Figure 5.25, the host-cell nucleus is caught at the moment of ejection. Microgametocytes (Figures 5.25, 5.26) have pale-staining cytoplasm and a scattering of round, black pigment granules, and their diameter is usually about 7 μm. This was found to be the average diameter of circular microgametocytes of *P. relictum* ssp. *capistranoae* as studied in Hawaiian Honeycreepers (Family Fringillidae, Tribe Drepanidini) by Laird and van Riper (1981). Just as in *P. matutinum*, both male and female gametocytes of *P. relictum* ssp. *capistranoae* are commonly present at the centre of enucleated host cells (see Laird and van Riper 1981, figures 14 and 15). Their overall resemblance in the two taxa, both in their adverse effects upon the host-cell nucleus and their size and morphology, is striking. Indeed, the only significant difference concerns the pigment granules. While similarly scattered and commonly numbering 10–15 in both species, these are characteristically round in *P. matutinum* but tend to include cone-shaped and somewhat cylindrical granules among the spherical ones in *P. relictum* ssp. *capistranoae* as pointed out by Russell (1932b).

Comparison of the schizonts of the latter parasite with those of the former is equally enlightening. In both the host cell tends to become rounded as development proceeds, the parasite pigment becoming conspicuously clumped (see the data and illustrations herein and Garnham 1966, figure 4, plate XLIV). Moreover, the range of merozoite number for *P. relictum* ssp. and *P. matutinum* is much the same, with good evidence of fluctuating averages as between host species, as might be expected where different strains from different avian hosts are concerned. Again, Russell (1932b) referred to vacuolation of the developing schizonts of his parasite as being not uncommon. Vacuoles were usually conspicuous in both the present MAPS infections from the type host at Dalton Pass, Philippines (p. 34), and in MAPS *P. matutinum* (Figure 5.3). The large, circular vacuoles of the latter species were aptly described as "punched out" by Garnham (1966) and convincingly illustrated by him and in the photomicrographs of Italian slides in Corradetti, Neri and Scanga (1960). While such vacuoles have not been reported from *P. relictum* ssp. *capistranoae*, they were, however, common among the heavier *P. matutinum* infections from several of its MAPS hosts (Table 5.3), that is, *Treron curvirostra, Lanius cristatus, L. validirostris, Copsychus saularis, Luscinia cyane, Zosterops japonicus, Trichastoma rostratum* and *Ploceus philippinus*. Garnham (1966) rates highest among the morphological features differentiating *P. matutinum* from *P. relictum* **s.l.**, "the presence of the characteristic vacuoles in all stages of the parasite except the gametocyte and mature schizont, *but this feature may not be marked in all strains*" [italics added by author].

That last phrase highlights the very real difficulty of differentiating between most species of subgenus *Haemamoeba* from field-collected blood smears unsupported by laboratory experimentation. The problem is particularly marked as between *P. matutinum* and *P. relictum* ssp. *capistranoae*, and would be further compounded were these to be synonymized, as the latter name would then have priority. As matters stand, a morphologically based decision in favour of *P. matutinum* must rest on evidence of synchronicity; which is of course not to be had in chronic infections with low parasitaemia. In such infections "*Plasmodium* sp?" must often be the only resort. Bearing in mind that 16 (37%) of MAPS hosts for *P. matutinum* were Brown Shrikes, *Lanius cristatus*, it thus seems likely that at least some of the 26 birds of this species shown as hosts for *Plasmodium* sp.? (Table 3.1) really harboured this parasite. Synchronicity was, however, detectable in all *L. cristatus* and other hosts listed in Table 5.3 as positive for *P. matutinum*.

Plasmodium (Haemamoeba) giovannolai Corradetti, Verolini and Neri 1963 (?)

Another *Haemamoeba* characterized by a 24 h schizogonic cycle and synchronicity, *P. giovannolai* was described from a Eurasian Blackbird, *Turdus merula* Linnaeus 1758 [WN 761.1], taken alive near Rome. On transfer to laboratory canaries the parasite not only showed a high level of synchronicity, but also its exoerythrocytic schizonts in the spleen proved much larger than those of other species of *Haemamoeba*, measuring up to 38.4 × 12 μm and producing 300+ merozoites (Corradetti, Verolini and Neri 1963). These authors stressed the invasion of erythroblasts, both polychromatophils and those with the cytoplasm still basophilic. Multiple invasions by trophozoites were extremely common so that individual cells came to contain seven or eight trophozoites.

The earliest of these were described as solid bodies of a micron in diameter. Colour plate 1, figure 6 of Corradetti, Verolini and Neri (1963) shows a young red cell containing six older trophozoites of irregular (somewhat polygonal) shape. Each has a conspicuous chromatin mass and an irregular vacuole bordered on three of its sides by a thick strand of cytoplasm. An inconspicuous black pigment granule appears as trophozoites age. More such granules become evident, as do one or more small vacuoles, as division begins. The host-cell nuclear displacement and tilting common to all members of the subgenus *Haemamoeba* is then well-advanced. Mature schizonts exhibit 10–30 (average 18) nuclei, their pigment granules coalescing into an off-centre or peripheral mass. Corradetti, Verolini and Neri (1963) stated that the spherical or spheroidal gametocytes are "con caratteri indistinguibili da quelli di *P. praecox* o di *P. matutinum*" [with characters indistinguishable from those of *P. praecox* or of *P. matutinum*]. However, there is a point of difference from these, for although both mature schizonts and mature gametocytes of *P. giovannolai* displace the host-cell nucleus to a side or pole of the cell, nuclear ejection has not been reported.

A Clamorous Reed-Warbler, *Acrocephalus stentoreus*, from which a blood smear was made at Mahárlú, Iran, (Eurasian–African Temperate Subregion) on 25 June 1967, proved to be very heavily parasitized by a *Plasmodium* of subgenus *Haemamoeba*. It exhibited up to 10 or 12 invaded cells — all of them immature erythrocytes, and usually some with basophilic cytoplasm — per oil immersion (×15) field of view. Virtually all plasmodia seen were freshly invaded merozoites to early trophozoites. Otherwise, 3 h of continuous scanning revealed only three segmenters with 20, 28 and 30 separating merozoites. The latter were condensed to the customary diameter (about 1.0 μm) of just-invaded merozoites/earliest trophozoites (Corradetti, Verolini and Neri 1963). In all three instances the host-cell nucleus was radically displaced.

Several just-invaded merozoites in immature red cells of *Acrocephalus stentoreus* are evident in Figure 5.28. Three in the corpuscle to left of the scale-line show no trace of cytoplasm. That corpuscle also contains irregularly shaped trophozoites at the earliest stage of development, the single chromatin mass and thick thread of cytoplasm surrounding the vacuole clearly evident. Additional merozoites had obviously continued to invade the cell following the initial invasion. Two cells to the right is a young erythrocyte containing three trophozoites, two of them at the first post-merozoite stage with a central vacuole.

Above these tiny "signet rings" is the result of a slightly earlier invasion, an irregular parasite in which the first chromatin division has initiated the early schizont stage. The nuclei of the two cells containing the above young parasites, are still located in the normal position. That of a third cell, with basophilic cytoplasm, some 17 mm above the right end of the scale-bar, is slightly displaced laterally.

Figure 5.29 was photographed from a blood slide from *Acrocephalus aedon*, the Thick-billed Warbler. It shows a developing schizont of *P. giovannolai*, with 14 nuclei and two or three granules of black pigment that have not yet clumped. The host-cell nucleus is radically displaced to the cell periphery, as is usual at this stage of development of species of the subgenus *Haemamoeba*. This was the only schizont found in a 45 min search by oil immersion. However, young red cells containing up to eight recently invaded merozoites and early trophozoites, exactly like those described above, were common. A few examples of a species of *Haemoproteus* accompanying the *P. giovannolai* infection had faded quite badly. This was probably referable to *Haemoproteus wenyoni* de Mello *et al.* (emend. Bennett, Bishop and Peirce 1991).

Points in favour of this *Plasmodium* being *P. giovannolai* are as follows. First, the sheer weight of the multiple invasion of immature red cells in the Iranian infection — a count of 300 parasitized cells revealed 40 (13.3%) with one recently invaded merozoite or very early trophozoite; 36 (12%) with 2; 26 (8.7%) with 3; 28 (9.3%) with 4; 36 (12%) with 5; 28 (9.3%) with 6; 33 (11%) with 7; 29 (9.7%) with 8; 17 (5.7%) with 9; 13 (4.3%) with 10; 6 (2%) with 11; and 8 (2.7%) with 12. Moreover, the very few phagocytes present had their cytoplasm rich in ingested merozoites. Presumably others, having reached full capacity, had left the peripheral circulation. As already mentioned, 3 h of (oil immersion) searching revealed only three segmenters on this slide. Failing actual laboratory experimentation, this combination of circumstances provided all the evidence that a blood smear can, of an extremely high degree of synchronicity. Furthermore, the morphology of the early trophozoites is precisely as described and illustrated by Corradetti, Verolini and Neri (1963) for *P. giovannolai*. Also both the nature of the red cells attacked and their impact upon those cells is in accordance with these authors' data. Last, the frequency of multiple invasion agrees with, and is even more striking than in, the original description; for the highest number of invading merozoites and early trophozoites seen in a single host cell by Corradetti, Verolini and Neri (1963) was eight. However, although 9 to 12 were attained in the Iranian infection, 85.3% of the 300 host cells from which counts were made held eight or less parasites. The incidences at the top end of the register were obviously tailing off, with 2% for 11 and 2.7% for 12. The displacement of host-cell nuclei by the very few mature schizonts seen, was as described by Corradetti, Verolini and Neri (1963).

Turning to the *Acrocephalus aedon* infection from Thailand, multiple infections at the commencement of the asexual cycle did not exceed the eight mentioned in the original description of *P. giovannolai*. The finding of but one schizont was in keeping with a highly synchronous cycle.

Points against identifying this malaria parasite as *P. giovannolai* must now be considered. First, no gametocytes were seen in either infection. Even though the sexual stages of all taxa of the subgenus *Haemamoeba* are rather alike, except for those of *P. cathemerium* characterized by spindle-shaped pigment granules, an absence of gametocytes from the MAPS parasite cannot preclude their having significant features of difference from *P. giovannolai*. Second, the duration of schizogony remains unknown. Third, the exceptionally high incidence of multiple invasions of erythroblasts, while strongly suggestive of *P. giovannolai*, may not altogether rule out some other member of subgenus *Haemamoeba*. However, its asynchronous schizogonic cycle eliminates *P. relictum* from further comparison. *P. subpraecox* is unknown from natural hosts other than Strigidae, and the lack of reports of more than six invasive merozoites/early trophozoites in *P. cathemerium* suggests that this species was not in question either. In any case, the failure to find any gametocytes in the MAPS material under consideration would preclude its positive identification as *P. cathemerium* because of the latter's key distinguishing feature in blood smears, the spindle-shaped pigment granules of microgametocytes. *P. gallinaceum*, being known with certainty only from *Gallus gallus*, is an unlikely candidate too, despite up to ten early asexual stages having been reported per host cell on occasion. This leaves only the asynchronous *P. relictum* ssp. *capistranoae* and the highly synchronous *P. matutinum*, with its precise 24 h periodicity. From the available evidence, the latter seems a far less likely determination for the *Acrocephalus* parasite than *P. giovannolai*, as multiple invasions of *P. matutinum* appear limited to 3–4 merozoites/early trophozoites per host cell.

Weighing the above for and against an identification of *P. giovannolai*, and while recognizing that there is a good case in favour of such a decision, it is concluded that the lack of anything approaching an adequate range of schizonts and of any gametocytes at all precludes more than a "possible" determination. Nevertheless, the previous lack of reports of this parasite east of Italy is not felt to be added reason for rejecting the possibility out of hand. Both the type host, *Turdus merula* and the MAPS host (*Acrocephalus stentoreus*) from which the most intriguing range of material was obtained, are long-range migrants which nest in the Palaearctic and winter in India and Southeast Asia (McClure 1974). *Acrocephalus aedon* is migratory too, and migration stress is well known to be productive of relapse in avian *Haemospororina* — notably *Leucocytozoon* as well as *Plasmodium* (Laird and Bennett 1970). Such birds might be expected to exhibit unusually high incidence of these haematozoa in their peripheral circulation while breaking their journey en route to or from breeding grounds. They might also act as reservoirs of infection for appropriate vectors able to spread the parasites to non-immune local hosts.

6

Plasmodium (Giovannolaia)

Plasmodium (Giovannolaia) fallax Schwetz 1930

Probably seen in the first decade of this century in East African Guineafowls (Garnham 1966), *P. fallax* was much later described from a typical owl (Strigidae) in today's Zaire — or as of May 1997, once again the Democratic Republic of Congo. It remains best known from this family, which was its only source during the present investigation. Other reports include that of Greiner and Mundy (1979) from *Gyps [bengalensis] africanus* Salvadori 1865, the White-backed Vulture [WN 6041], sampled in Zimbabwe.

Garnham (1966) declared that asexual schizogony in *P. fallax* "is so asynchronous that the duration of the cycle in the blood has not been determined". He remarked that the merozoites, which Huff *et al.* (1960) found to be distinctly curved, usually invade mature erythrocytes, that ring-form trophozoites are rare, and that developing trophozoites soon exhibit one or two "curiously white", circular vacuoles. Garnham recognized the possibility of confusing these with the volutin granules of young haemoproteids. Bishop and Bennett (1989) explained that such granules can appear dark blue or purple or show as clear vacuoles, depending on the intensity of the Romanowsky stain used. Such "curiously white", circular vacuoles were evident in small, polar trophozoites of a Collared Scops-Owl from Nakhon Ratchasima, Thailand, that was also parasitized by *P. relictum* ssp. *relictum* but lacked haemoproteids. As growth proceeds, occasional filiform pseudopodia are seen projecting from both trophozoites and early schizonts, as mentioned by Garnham (1966). Always diminutive, these never approached the size of the ones so characteristic of *P. (Giovannolaia) dissanaikei*, and they were only seen in *Otus lempiji*. Nine birds of four species yielded *P. fallax* in the MAPS material (Table 6.1).

Developing schizonts tend to be positioned laterally to the host-cell nucleus, which is occasionally somewhat pushed aside but seldom as far as the cell membrane (Figure 6.1). This figure displays the relatively

Table 6.1 Findings of ***Plasmodium (Giovannolaia) fallax***

Host species[1] (individual positive records)	Associated haematozoa[2]	Localities	Months
Ninox philippensis	*H. syrnii, P.r.*	Basay, Negros Oriental, Philippines	December
Ninox philippensis	*H. noctuae, P.r.r.*	Negros, Philippines	November
Otus lempiji	*H. noctuae*	Ban Chiang Dao, Thailand	October
Otus lempiji	*H. syrnii*	Nakhon Ratchasima, Thailand	September
Otus lempiji	*P.r.r.*	Nakhon Ratchasima, Thailand	September
Otus lempiji	*H. noctuae*	Nakhon Ratchasima, Thailand	September
Otus lempiji	*H. noctuae, P.n.*, mf	Chiang Mai, Thailand	October
Otus sunia	*H. syrnii, P.r.*	Sara Buri, Thailand	January
Otus spilocephalus	*H, L*	Chiang Mai, Thailand	February
Totals 4 host species	9 individuals +ve *P. fallax*		

[1] Taxonomic order as in Table 2.2.

[2] *Haemoproteus (H,* with species name where possible), *Leucocytozoon (L), Plasmodium* [*P. relictum* ssp. *relictum (P.r.r.); P. rouxi (P.r.); P. nucleophilum (P.n.)*] and microfilariae (mf).

large merozoite-precursors, measuring <1.4 μm in diameter. In mature schizonts, which stretch for some two-thirds to the full length of the red cell, three to six brownish pigment granules with a yellowish to golden glint are clumped near an extremity. A circular, whitish vacuole, larger than that of some trophozoites, may be adjacent. The range in merozoite number was 12–20 (av. 16). Garnham gave 18 as the upper limit. Greiner and Mundy (1979) specified 20 in material from *Gyps africanus*, from which their figure 3 illustrates a developing gametocyte with scattered pigment granules and bright little vacuoles as described by Garnham (1966) and seen in Figure 6.2 herein. In the latter the host-cell nucleus is somewhat displaced laterally, but not quite to the cell membrane. As described by Garnham (1966), mature gametocytes are unmistakable in having one end hooked around the scarcely displaced host-cell nucleus as in the microgametocytes of Figures 6.3 and 6.4a from *Otus lempiji*, Thailand, and *Ninox philippensis*, Negros Oriental, Philippines. These two figures show the typically vacuolated and pale-staining cytoplasm of the microgametocyte, with the scattered brownish pigment granules evident in Figure 6.3. A vacuolated but much darker staining macrogametocyte, with its heavily staining nucleus at the inner curve, is shown in Figure 6.4b, from the same preparation as Figure 6.4a. Nine to 16 pigment granules were counted in microgametocytes less heavily stained than the one illustrated. *P. fallax* gametocytes with irregularly crenate extremities were noticed among the different hosts.

In the only instance of a double invasion of a host erythrocyte encountered in the MAPS material, a developing schizont of *P. fallax* was tangentially positioned against one end of the host-cell nucleus. The latter was not displaced, and between one of its sides and the cell membrane the available space was occupied by a young haemoproteid with a conspicuous volutin granule, presumably *Haemoproteus noctuae* (as redescribed by Bishop and Bennett 1989). Circumnuclear gametocytes of this haemoproteid were present in a smear from Chiang Mai, Thailand (2 October 1967), exhibiting a quadruple infection of the haemoproteid, *P. fallax*, *P. (Novyella) nucleophilum* and a single microfilaria (Table 6.1) in the Collared Scops-Owl.

These are the first "justified" identifications of *P. fallax* from the Asian Tropical Subregion. However, three of the Thai *Otus lempiji* (formerly *O. bakkamoena*)records, and that from *O. spilocephalus*, were mentioned without taxonomic data by McClure *et al.* (1978). Otherwise, previous reports (see host-parasite catalogues of Bennett, Whiteway and Woodworth–Lynas 1982; Bennett *et al.* 1992) concern Africa only.

Plasmodium (Giovannolaia) circumflexum Kikuth 1931

This species was described from Germany, although believed to have been encountered elsewhere in Europe and North America long before (Garnham 1966). Garnham cited findings from Morocco, Brazil, Bangladesh and Sri Lanka. There was also a likely misidentification of it from *Ardeola (ralloides) grayii* (Sykes) 1832 [WN 2038], the Indian Pond Heron (Basu 1938). Garnham considered *Plasmodium circumflexum* to be "largely confined to passerine birds" and summed up its tropical distribution as patchy. Subsequent investigations have disproved both statements — Bennett, Whiteway and Woodworth-Lynas (1982) listing numerous findings from non-passerines as well as from tropical countries.

All six MAPS records of *P. circumflexum* were, however, from passerines (Table 6.2). Four were from three species of *Pycnonotus* (bulbuls), the single previous report from this genus being that of Bennett, Okia and Cameron (1974). Only two findings were from Malaysia as compared with Ogaki's (1949) World War II 33 *P. circumflexum* records from there. Ogaki's overall total of birds sampled was only 198 as compared with the MAPS figure of 55 289. This could be interpreted as supporting

Table 6.2 Findings of ***Plasmodium (Giovannolaia) circumflexum***

Host species[1] (individual positive records)	Associated haematozoa[2]	Localities	Months
Oriolus chinensis	*H. P.v.*, mf	Siaton, Negros, Philippines	November
Sturnus nigricollis	*H. pastoris, P.n.*	Bang Phra, Cholburi, Thailand	December
Pycnonotus goiavier	–	Kuala Pisang, Malaysia	July
Pycnonotus goiavier	*L. P.d.*	Bang Phra, Cholburi, Thailand	October
Pycnonotus melanoleucos	*P.v.*	Sakaerat, Pakthong Chai, Thailand	June
Pycnonotus simplex	*H. octocompsae, P.m.*	Subang, Malaysia	July

Totals 5 host species and 6 individuals +ve *P. circumflexum*

[1] Taxanomic order as in Table 2.2.

[2] *Haemoproteus* (*H*, with species name where possible), *Leucocytozoon (L.)*, *Plasmodium* [*P. matutinum (P.m.)*; *P. dissanaikei (P.d.)*; *P. vaughani (P.v.)*; *P. nucleophilum (P.n.)*] and microfilariae (mf).

Garnham's (1966) statement that "Records of the species made by the Japanese in Malaya at the end of the Second World War are doubtful". Alternatively, it might suggest that formerly effective mosquito control measures had utterly broken down in the aftermath of invasion and conquest, and that consequent flourishing of vectors had triggered a pandemic of *P. circumflexum*-induced avian malaria. In either event, it is of interest that none of the five species of Malaysian birds recorded by Ogaki (1949) as harbouring *P. circumflexum* proved positive for this parasite in the MAPS collections. Moreover, two of them, *Copsychus saularis* and *Lonchura punctulata*, were represented by as many as 862 and 349 examples, respectively, in the present material.

As in the Bangladesh strain of *P. circumflexum* from *Sturnus malabaricus* and *Acridotheres tristis* studied by Laird and Lari (1958), the other certain Asian Tropical Subregion strains from six MAPS hosts all initially invaded polychromatophil erythroblasts and normoblasts. Multiple invasions of host cells by up to five merozoites occurred. The first chromatin division of the developing schizont takes place when the parasite attains the length of the host-cell nucleus (see Garnham 1966). In an example from *Sturnus nigricollis* advancing to the second such division, the schizont was scarcely larger. However, its chromatin formed two knob-terminated strands. By the third division, the schizonts were much longer than the host-cell nucleus (Figure 6.5). Vacuoles were appearing in their cytoplasm, and eight irregularly shaped chromatin masses were present. The sinuously margined octonucleate schizonts of *P. circumflexum* then had their chromatin masses in linear series, as illustrated by Laird and Lari (1958). Each such mass was destined for a final division, resulting in the formation of 16 merozoites. Other schizonts with only five or six large nuclei were likewise to divide once more, forming 10 or 12 merozoites.

Just as in the above Bangladesh material, the host-cell nucleus was often laterally displaced by now, through pressure from the schizont, swelling to fill the space between the nucleus and the cell membrane to one side of it (Figure 6.6). The ends of the schizont were now curved about those of the host-cell nucleus (the mid-line of the parasite of Figure 6.6 measured about 13.9 μm, as compared with the erythrocyte's 12.5 μm length). These dimensions compared closely with those of Laird and Lari (1958) from Bangladesh *Acridotheres tristis*, in which erythrocyte length averaged 13.6 μm, the mid-line length of schizonts averaging 14.7 μm. The longest schizont mid-line measurement from MAPS material was 16.4 μm, in a 15.3 μm-long corpuscle of the Bang Phra *Sturnus nigricollis*.

From the earliest schizonts onwards, dark brown to yellowish-golden pigment granules were massed near an extremity. Towards segmentation, from three to seven (av. 4) of these granules could still be distinguished in such clumps. As the large (<1.5 μm) merozoites dispersed, so did these granules. Fading readily as the stained blood films aged, none remained evident when the photomicrographs were taken; but pigment was always prominent in sketches made when the slides were still fresh. Few schizonts "entirely girdling the nucleus" were seen (Garnham 1966). Nevertheless, occasional mature ones (Figures 6.7, 6.8) occupied most of the intracorpuscular space, the host-cell nucleus becoming displaced towards the cell membrane. Heavily stained, tightly packed merozoites could only be counted with difficulty.

More than 16 were certainly present in the segmenter of Figure 6.7. The small, circular vacuoles persist until segmentation (Figure 6.8). At segmentation there were 8–24 merozoites. The numbers for *Oriolus chinensis* were 10–16, *Sturnus nigricollis* 10–22, *Pycnonotus goiavier* 8–18, *P. melanoleucos* 12–24 and *P. simplex* 10–18.

All the MAPS field infections were clearly chronic ones. There were inadequate numbers of segmenters for meaningful averages to be obtained. However, the usual merozoite counts were within the 12/14/16 range, as was the case for a heavy (laboratory) infection in Bangladesh *Sturnus malabaricus* in which the following results (Table 6.3) from 100 successive segmenters are from Laird and Lari (1958):

Table 6.3 Heavy (laboratory) infection in Bangladesh *Sturnus malabaricus*; results from 100 successive segmenters (Laird and Lari 1958)

Merozoites	Percentage
10	3
12	27
14	40
16	21
18	5
20	2
22	1
24	1

One *Sturnus malabaricus* schizont from Bangladesh had 26 nuclei (Laird and Lari 1958).

The highest count from the MAPS *P. circumflexum* material was of 24 separated merozoites, evenly distributed about the still-centrally positioned nucleus of a *Pycnonotus melanoleucos* erythrocyte. Garnham (1966) gave the overall merozoite range in *P. circumflexum* as 6–30, warning that "double infections may give rise to miscalculation of the real merozoite number". There was no danger of confusion in the MAPS instances, for a single conspicuous group of pigment granules was always free in the red cell together with the merozoites. When separated but still within the host cell, and afterwards when free in the plasma, merozoites were oval to elongate and slightly crescentic (Laird and Lari 1958, figures 14–17a); the latter type measuring some 2.0×0.9 μm in their greatest dimensions.

Freehand sketches made when the material was first received show both immature and mature gametocytes typical of this species. The former curved around both poles of the host-cell nucleus, somewhat displacing it laterally. Mature gametocytes completely surrounded the host-cell nucleus, which was not appreciably displaced — having roughly equal thicknesses of the gametocyte on either side. When freshly stained, macrogametocytes of MAPS *P. circumflexum* exhibited about 20 dark brown, scattered pigment granules, varying in size and of oval or spherical shape. Their nucleus was rose-staining, large and approximately central in examples that had only curved about the poles of the host-cell nucleus. It was diffuse and pinkish in microgametocytes. This stage of the parasite conformed to earlier descriptions, and in particular to Bangladesh material (Laird and Lari 1958, figures 19–22). Laird and Lari's figure 19 shows a gametocyte very like the faded one seen in Figure 6.9 herein, which, however, is *Haemoproteus pastoris* (de Mello 1936; emend. Bishop and Bennett 1990).

MAPS *P. circumflexum* were easily separated from other Haemospororina, the only real possibility of confusion concerning the accompanying representative of its own subgenus, *P. dissanaikei* (Chapter 6, pp. 63–67) in the Bang Phra infection from *Pycnonotus goiavier* (Table 6.2). While the earliest stages would be difficult to separate, older trophozoites and developing schizonts of *P. dissanaikei* on the slide exhibited this species' characteristic filopodia. Moreover, *P. dissanaikei* segmenters never have more than 12 merozoites, and do not surround the poles of the host-cell nucleus; and the latter is never totally encircled by this parasite's gametocytes. Finally, in the *Pycnonotus simplex* triple infection (Table 6.2) the thick, semihalteridial gametocytes of *Haemoproteus octocompsae* are quite unlike the sexual stages of the associated *P. circumflexum* and *P. matutinum*. One of three species of *Haemoproteus* now recognized from the Pycnonotidae, it has already been recorded from MAPS *Pycnonotus simplex* by Rahal, Bishop and Bennett (1986).

Plasmodium (Giovannolaia) polare Manwell 1934

Plasmodium polare was described from (*Petrochelidon lunifrons*) = *Hirundo pyrrhonota* (Vieillot) 1817, the Cliff Swallow [WN 612], from Westport, New York, USA (Manwell 1934; 1935b). Cassamagnagli (1945a;b; 1947a;b) reported it from tinamous in Uruguay, and Ray *et al.* (1953) claimed to have identified it from an Indian phasianid, *Francolinus pondicerianus* (Gmelin) 1789, the Grey Francolin [WN 288.4]. Theirs was a likely description of a species of the subgenus *Giovannolaia* (*G. dissanaikei*?) but as Garnham (1966) recognized, one unlikely to be *P. polare*; other records of which are from, for example, American doves (Al-Dabagh 1964) and sparrows (Bennett, Whiteway and Woodworth-Lynas 1982), and from Europe's Common Kestrel [WN 359.1], *Falco (tinnunculus) tinnunculus*, from which Corradetti and Scanga (1963; 1965) published a good account of it from Sicilian material. Otherwise, Garnham's (1966) reference to *P. polare* as an "apparently rare parasite" was still justified a quarter of a century ago.

Since then, though, this species has been identified from additional passerine hosts in both North and South America (Bennett, Whiteway and Woodworth-Lynas 1982), in former Czechoslovakia (Kucera 1978) and in Asian republics of the former USSR (see p. 60). Various additional birds have been added to its host-list in recent years. These include kestrels (Tadzhikistan: Subkhonov 1972a), eagles (Florida, USA: Greiner, Black and Iverson 1981) and ducks (New Brunswick, Canada: Meyer and Bennett 1976; Tchad: Williams, Bennett and Troncy 1977). The last-mentioned record, with passerine ones from Senegal and southern Africa (Bennett *et al.* 1978; Bennett, Whiteway and Woodworth-Lynas 1982) were the first for *P. polare* from tropical Africa.

P. polare can thus no longer be termed uncommon. To date, though, the only published records of its occurrence in the Asian Tropical Subregion have been the erroneous one of Ray *et al.* (1953) from India already mentioned, and unsupported preliminary mentions (Laird 1966; Laird and Grewal 1968; McClure *et al.* 1978) of some of the MAPS material now listed and discussed herein.

Despite the claim of Corradetti and Scanga (1963) that *P. polare* exhibits a 24 h periodicity, an overview of collective experience (based largely on blood slides alone) counsels that "the density of parasitaemia is too low for the determination of the duration of schizogony" (Garnham 1966). The earliest stages have seldom been illustrated elsewhere than close to one of the poles of the invaded cell.

The 27 infections studied in 17 avian species from the MAPS collections (Table 6.4) were chronic, and without any evidence of tightly synchronous periodicity of the asexual cycle. Mature schizonts with a few segmenters exhibiting dispersing merozoites were quite common in the second Malaysian slide from *Anthreptes malacensis*. A single corpuscle containing two polar merozoites was seen. An early trophozoite level with a tip of the undisturbed host-cell nucleus was noticed in the slide from the February example of *Trichastoma rostratum* from Rantau Panjang, and a laterally placed signet-ring stage resembling that illustrated in plate VIII of Hewitt (1940) was sketched from the September preparation of *Otus lempiji* from Sabah (Table 6.4). The same slide yielded polar schizonts in the earliest stage of nuclear division, with two to four granules of dark brown pigment.

Figure 6.10 illustrates a tangentially placed, elongate trophozoite from *Pycnonotus melanicterus* in a polar location. The development and maturation of the schizont of *P. polare* typically proceed at one end of the cell, where the available space is largely filled soon after the commencement of nuclear division (Figure 6.11). The illustration shows the relative abundance of cytoplasm at that stage, a feature that serves to distinguish *P. polare* from the equivalent stage of *P. (Novyella) vaughani* with which it was sometimes associated.

Figure 6.12 illustrates the penultimate chromatin division of a *P. polare* schizont in the uncommon latero/polar location for this species shown by some earlier authors (e.g. Hewitt 1940; Garnham 1966). The schizont of Figure 6.12 has unusually large nuclei, and relatively little cytoplasm. Its pigment is hidden by the six chromatin masses. These are pyriform, reflecting internal pressures exerted during nuclear division in fan-shaped (or in this instance, butterfly-shaped) schizonts. Such schizonts are far more characteristic of the subgenus *Novyella* in general, and *P. vaughani* in particular, than of *P. polare*.

The former parasite was associated with *P. polare* in the preparation just mentioned. Although neither was common, a representative range

Table 6.4 Findings of ***Plasmodium (Giovannolaia) polare***

Host species[1] (individual positive records)	Associated haematozoa[2]	Localities	Months
Turnix suscitator	*P.v.*	Kuala Lumpur, Malaysia	April
Turnix suscitator	*P.v.*	Kuala Lumpur, Malaysia	December
Turnix suscitator	*T*	Palawan, Philippines	May
Megalaima asiatica	*H. cornuata*	Chiang Mai, Thailand	December
Megalaima chrysopogon	–	Sabah, E. Malaysia	?
Todirhamphus chloris	*H. halcyonis*	Negros, Philippines	April
Otus lempiji	*T*	Sabah, E. Malaysia	September
Otus lempiji	*H. syrnii, P.r.*	Subang, E. Malaysia	June
Otus spilocephalus	*H. syrnii*	Mt Brinchang, Malaysia	February
Otus sunia	–	Southern Thailand	October
Amaurornis phoenicurus	*P.r.* ***s.l.***	Rantau Panjang, Malaysia	April
Amaurornis phoenicurus	*P.r.*	Rantau Panjang, Malaysia	April
Amaurornis phoenicurus	–	Rantau Panjang, Malaysia	April
Amaurornis phoenicurus	–	Subang, Malaysia	November
Lanius cristatus	*H. lanii, P.m.*	Subang, Malaysia	September
Dicrurus annectans	*P.v.*	Subang, Malaysia	October
Dicrurus balicassius	–	Palawan, Philippines	February
Dicrurus balicassius	mf	Basay, Negros Oriental, Philippines	December
Dicrurus balicassius	*H,L, P.v., At*	Basay, Negros Oriental, Philippines	December
Pycnonotus melanicterus	*T, L*	Mt Brinchang, Malaysia	March
Pycnonotus squamatus	*L*, mf	Kuala Pisang, Malaysia	July
Trichastoma rostratum	–	Rantau Panjang, Malaysia	October
Trichastoma rostratum	*P.r.*	Rantau Panjang, Malaysia	February
Anthreptes malacensis	*H. sequeirae*	Rantau Panjang, Malaysia	April
Anthreptes malacensis	*H. sequeirae*	Rantau Panjang, Malaysia	?
Nectarinia jugularis	*P.m.*	Tarabanan, Palawan, Philippines	May
Ploceus philippinus	–	Sungei Way, Malaysia	January
Totals	17 host species and 27 individuals +ve *P. polare*		

[1] Taxonomic order as in Table 2.2.

[2] *Trypanosoma (T), Haemoproteus (H,* with species name where possible), *Leucocytozoon (L), Plasmodium [P. relictum* ***sensu lato*** *(P.r.s.l.); P. matutinum (P.m.), P. vaughani (P.v.), P. rouxi (p.r.)], Atoxoplasma (At)* and microfilariae (mf).

of schizonts was present for both. However, there was little difficulty in differentiating the two species. The chromatin masses of *P. polare* at the penultimate division stage (Figures 6.12, 6.13) measured about 1.4 × 1.1 μm, but those of *P. vaughani* (in similar fan configurations, or in the cruciform or box-formation ones usual when only four merozoites result) never exceed 1.0 μm in their greatest dimension (Figure 6.14a,b). Furthermore, the chromatin masses of hexanucleate schizonts of *P. vaughani* tend to average only about 0.8 μm in their greatest dimension. When consolidated and dispersed, the merozoites of the latter parasite range in diameter from about 0.5 to 0.7 μm when six result (Figure 6.15), and from about 0.3 to 0.5 μm when eight are formed (Figure 6.16). The apparent triviality of these measurements disappears on comparison of the hexanucleate penultimate division stage of a

P. polare schizont (Figure 6.12) with the hexanucleate *P. vaughani* segmenter of Figure 6.14b. Comparisons between younger schizonts are instructive too. Note the far greater size (6.1 × 4.5 μm) of *P. polare* (Figure 6.11) compared with that of *P. vaughani* (3.3 × 2.4 μm) in Figure 6.17; and also, the deeper staining and less vacuolated cytoplasm of *P. polare*.

Because of the intensely staining chromatin of the *P. polare* polar schizont of Figure 6.13, the nuclear number is not clear in the photomicrograph. However, with oil immersion and intense transmitted light, eight chromatin masses could be counted. The cytoplasm of this maturing schizont, which was destined to form 16 merozoites, is relatively far more evident than that of the putative octonucleate segmenter (with a large chromatin mass still to complete division, at top) of *P. vaughani* seen in Figure 6.16. Also, the assertiveness of the dark brown pigment mass at the tip of the "handle" of an octonucleate fan of *P. polare* in Figure 6.13 is strikingly different from the dot-like equivalent granule arrowed in Figure 6.18.

The six chromatin masses of the irregular polar schizont of Figure 6.19 were each destined to divide again. This schizont's appearance — down to the bright little vacuoles, indicative of more cytoplasm than ever characterizes *P. vaughani* — closely compares with that of *P. polare* from the Common Kestrel illustrated in photomicrograph 4 of Corradetti and Scanga (1963). Figure 6.20 shows a unique feature of the latter parasite stressed by Garnham (1966). This is the "peculiar 'stranded' appearance" of segmenters with 8–14 large merozoites, the stranding due to thin threads of cytoplasm separating still-persisting vacuoles. Figure 6.21 shows the end result of segmentation for an octonucleate schizont of the fan-type seen in Figure 6.13. While the densely stained and still-crowded merozoites appear to number six in the photomicrograph, eight could be differentiated in bright-field microscopy (no trace of either cytoplasm or pigment was then seen). Advocates of the validity of "*P. hexamerium*" (now generally considered a synonym of *P. vaughani*, see p. 69) might relegate the parasite of Figure 6.21 to the former, especially as Huff (1935), who proposed the name for a customarily six-nucleate avian malaria parasite, admitted its occasional formation of eight merozoites. The solitary report of "*P. hexamerium*" from the Asian Tropical Subregion (Manwell, Allen and Kuntz 1976) concerns Taiwan, and is discussed under *P. vaughani* (Chapter 7, p. 73). This species has never been associated with more than trifling displacement of the host-cell nucleus, which is pronounced in Figure 6.21. The degree of lateral displacement shown in the latter accords with that illustrated in examples of *P. polare* by Hewitt (1940), Corradetti and Scanga (1963) and Greiner, Black and Iverson (1981). Additional evidence for the true identity of the subject of Figure 6.21 comes from the common occurrence in *P. polare* of still larger, irregular schizonts with 10 (Figure 6.22), 12 or 14 condensing merozoites.

Twenty-four mature schizonts and segmenters selected at random from the entire MAPS sample of *P. polare* yielded the following counts: two instances of eight merozoites, 16 of 10, 4 of 12 and 2 of 14 (av. 10.5). This accords with Garnham's (1966) analysis, indicating a range of 8–14 (av. 10 or 11) in North American strains. Colombian figures (Ayala and

Varela 1975) were generally 8–12 (av. 10.2), with rare findings of six. The Sicilian Kestrel strain of this parasite appears to have a broader range of merozoite number. Corradetti and Scanga (1963) gave a range of 6–16 from both the natural host and laboratory canaries, but with 53% and 55% of the respective counts numbering eight and only 21% and 22% numbering 10.

Gametocytes of *P. polare* (Figures 6.23–6.25) extend the length of the host cell and usually curve somewhat about the poles of its nucleus. The larger ones cause some lateral displacement of the latter (Garnham 1966; see photomicrographs 11 and 12 of Corradetti and Scanga 1963 and photomicrograph 2 of Greiner, Black and Iverson 1981). Their superficial resemblance to *Haemoproteus* is obvious enough, but their often-ragged outline (Ayala and Varela 1975) militates against this. Thus the smoothly margined, immature gametocyte of *Haemoproteus sequeirae* (Tendeiro 1947; emend. Bennett, Peirce and Caines 1984) of Figure 6.26 is very different from the sexual stages of *P. polare*, with their far more irregular outline. Examples of the latter are seen in Figures 6.23 and 6.24. The first, a macrogametocyte with a finger-like projection from its uppermost end, closely resembles that (from the Sicilian strain of *P. polare*) seen in Garnham's (1966) figure 24, plate LI. The second, a microgametocyte of comparable size to the haemoproteid of Figure 6.26, sharply differs from the latter in its irregular outline and much more conspicuous vacuolation. These features also characterize the microgametocyte of Figure 6.25, with its conspicuous, centrally located nucleus. It has been suggested (Ayala and Varela 1975; Greiner, Black and Iverson 1981) that such ragged or scalloped gametocyte peripheries of *P. polare* indicate senescence. Evenly margined examples were also present in the smears examined by these workers, and in the MAPS material. While these are more easily confused with *H. sequeirae* at the stage shown in Figure 6.26, the mature forms of this haemoproteid differ from *P. polare* in curving about the ends of the host-cell nucleus in halteridial fashion (Bennett, Peirce and Caines 1984). None of the four other species of *Haemoproteus* associated with *P. polare* in MAPS smears (Table 6.4) had gametocytes likely to be confused with those of the latter.

P. polare is now known from numerous avian hosts of the Asian Tropical Subregion, from Negros, Philippines to Thailand (Table 6.4), with indications of a particularly heavy presence in Malaysia. As there are several recent reports from Tadzhikistan (Subkhonov 1972a) and Kazakhstan (Yakunin 1976; Yakunin and Zhazyltaev 1977; Kairullaev 1979), it seems likely that future trans-Himalayan bird migration studies concentrating on migratory species may reveal its presence in the Indian subcontinent and Myanmar (formerly Burma).

Plasmodium (Giovannolaia) lophurae Coggeshall 1938

The original and only laboratory strain of *P. lophurae* was isolated from a Bornean pheasant in the New York Zoological Park, its host, the Crested Fireback, being distinguished from the Malaysian ¶*rufa* (Raffles) 1822 under the name of Vieillot's Fireback, *Lophura ignita* ¶*ignita* (Shaw) 1797 [WN 3093]. Whether or not this was a natural host necessarily remained uncertain because of the possibility of the parasite having been acquired via an infective local mosquito vector that had previously bitten some other species of bird, whether endemic or exotic.

As no similar infections have been reported from the type locality or elsewhere in North America after more than half a century, *P. lophurae* must be assumed to have been imported with the type host. Its first mention from the Asian Tropical Subregion was that of Ogaki (1949). He claimed to have identified it from a single example of *Geopelia striata* in Kuala Lumpur, among 198 birds of seven species examined in Malaysia during the World War II Japanese occupation. His report, being unsubstantiated by morphological data, was questioned by Laird (1966). Another columbiform bird that is peridomestic, but far more widespread, the Rock Pigeon, *Columba livia*, has been shown to be a laboratory host for *P. lophurae*. Peridomestic columbiforms would, however, seem highly unlikely wild hosts for a haematozoan of which the only known natural host is a sylvatic phasianid.

The next field reports of *P. lophurae* were from Kazakhstan. Yakunin (1976) listed it there from *Sturnus vulgaris* and two species of *Emberiza*, both buntings being open-country birds, as is the Common Starling when not actually peridomestic. Ten further Kazakhstan hosts were added to these by Yakunin and Zhazyltaev (1977), two each in the Coraciiformes (a roller and a cuckoo), the Columbiformes (the Turtle Dove and Pale-backed Pigeon), the Ciconiiformes (the Sparrow Hawk and Montagu's Harrier) and the Passeriformes/Corvoidea (the Carrion Crow and Jackdaw); not to mention a bee-eater (Coraciiformes/Meropides) and a Brambling (Passeriformes/Passeri). These alleged findings shall be discussed after considering the taxonomic characters of *P. lophurae*.

P. lophurae has a decidedly asynchronous cycle in the blood. Some have thought schizogony had lasted for 36 h, although Garnham suggested 24 h as perhaps more likely. The following account of *P. lophurae* is based upon the only blood film from which this diagnosis was made in the entire MAPS project. The slide came from a single Crestless Fireback, *Lophura erythropthalma*, out of eight examined from lowland Malaysia. This forest bird was captured near Subang on 25 October 1962. Its infection was a chronic one, and accompanied by a few trophozoites and schizonts of an unidentified *Plasmodium*, (see p. 63; Figures 6.27, 6.28). Unlike *P. lophurae*, the latter caused marked displacement of the host-cell nucleus.

P. lophurae trophozoites were only found in mature erythrocytes of one of eight examples of *Lophura erythropthalma* that were sampled. Initially, solid polar and latero-polar examples were seen. Soon after the appearance of a central vacuole and a clearly brief signet-ring stage, the trophozoite's outline becomes irregular (Figure 6.29) and little filopodia develop. The vacuole remains large (about 1.7 μm) and bright. This was pointed out by Hewitt (1942), who found that panoptic staining rendered it pale orange. Figure 6.30 illustrates a developing schizont with horn-like filopodia at the upper end, and a tail-like pseudopod at the other (compare the second figure of the bottom sequence of Hewitt's (1940) plate VII). The author's and Hewitt's are both latero-polar. So is another such amoeboid late-trophozoite, in Garnham's figure 8, plate LIII, reproduced from Hewitt (1942). A schizont with unusually long terminal filopodia is seen in Figure 6.31.

Binary chromatin division is evident at the periphery of two prominent vacuoles in Figure 6.32. Noting that these vacuoles are colourless when Giemsa rather than panoptic staining is employed, Garnham (1966) felt them to be important diagnostic criteria for *P. lophurae*. Figure 6.33 shows a later stage in schizont development. Its cytoplasm exhibits smallish and no longer bright vacuoles. The dividing chromatin masses are heavily stained, a few grains of (dark brown) pigment have collected at the right end of the parasite, and there is only minor lateral displacement of the host-cell nucleus.

From this stage onwards, the nuclei of maturing schizonts of the Malaysian parasite number 8–18. The only segmenters identified had produced 18 (Figure 6.34a,b) and 10 (Figure 6.35) large merozoites. Those of Figure 6.34a are so closely crowded as to be uncountable in the illustration. By phase-contrast microscopy, though, using a green filter, the count was definitely 18. The 10 of Figure 6.35, being much less crowded, are evidently of the order of size characteristic of the subgenus *Giovannolaia*, their diameter approximating 1.7 μm. Garnham's review of the then-available (i.e. 1966) information, states that in *P. lophurae* "The mature schizont often has an elongated form, with minute grains of pigment concentrated into one or two areas. Eight to eighteen large merozoites are produced…" This exactly fits the parasites of Figures 6.34a,b and 6.35, in the last of which the single mass of dark brown pigment is arrowed. In Figure 6.34b a similar mass of pigment is obvious, having been brought out by filtering from the tight assemblage of merozoites obscuring it in Figure 6.34a.

Several elongate schizonts from the Malaysian Crestless Fireback were looped around an end of the host-cell nucleus, just as represented by Huff *et al.* (1947). Three of them had 14, 16 and 18 chromatin masses. They slightly displaced the erythrocyte nucleus longitudinally, and their 4–7 dot-like granules of dark brown pigment were clumped at an extremity. Three younger schizonts occasioned no nudging of the host-cell nucleus. Two were quadrinuculeate (Figures 6.31, 6.33), the other octonucleate (Figure 6.36). A single segmenter with dispersing merozoites (av. 1.3 μm) was seen. The host-cell nucleus remained central but was reduced in size and pyknotic. These merozoites were of similar size to those of *P. circumflexum* and, as in the latter parasite, were partially edged by cytoplasm.

Early figures of the sexual stages published soon after *P. lophurae* was described, represented both elongate gametocytes with slightly incurved extremities, and circumnuclear ones (Hewitt 1940; 1942). The few examples discovered in the Crestless Fireback smear were of the former type. There was occasional lateral displacement of the host-cell nucleus (Figure 6.37). This illustration also shows the conspicuous vacuolation of the macrogametocyte cytoplasm portrayed by Hewitt (1942). Although the pigment of the parasite of Figure 6.37 had faded when it was photographed, freshly stained macrogametocytes showed about ten oval granules scattered throughout the cytoplasm. Hewitt's (1940) plate VII, second-to-last sketch, illustrates a *P. lophurae* macrogametocyte with a finger-like terminal filopod resembling those of *P. polare* in Figure 6.23 herein and Garnham's (1966) plate LI, figure 24. Such filopodia characterize most representatives of *Giovannolaia*, and will be discussed at more length in pp. 55–56, being best developed in *P. dissanaikei*. Scalloping of the free outer margin of *P. lophurae* microgametocytes, as illustrated by Coggeshall (1938), is conspicuous in Figure 6.37. It was equally evident in another macrogametocyte, featuring two circular vacuoles, the larger being 2.6μm in diameter and spanning two-thirds of the organism's greatest width.

It is considered that the reports of *P. lophurae* from 13 species of passerine and other birds in Kazakhstan (p. 61) are as suspect as that of Ogaki (1949). Because of the close resemblances between *P. lophurae* and other species of subgenus *Giovannolaia* more likely to be found in central Asian hosts, and for ecological considerations (*Lophura* spp. are non-migratory birds of dense tropical forests), comparative morphological accounts and convincing illustrations are prerequisite to acceptance of these findings. Pending such data, the present account should stand as the first and only field record of *P. lophurae* from a natural host.

A few examples of a second species of *Plasmodium* accompanied *P. lophurae* in the Crestless Fireback slide. Unlike the latter parasite, it displaced and tilted the host-cell nucleus in *Haemamoeba*-like fashion (Figures 6.27, 6.28). The first of these illustrations shows two maturing octonucleate schizonts (line of demarcation arrowed) in a red cell. The octonucleate segmenter of Figure 6.28 has condensing merozoites measuring about 1.2–1.4 μm in diameter. Garnham (1966) found a very similar parasite in a Vieillot's Fireback that had died in the London Zoo. As shown in his plate LIII, figures 15–20, this also caused "marked displacement of the host-cell nucleus" once beyond the trophozoite stage. The octonucleate schizont of his figure 18 is so like that of Figure 6.28 here as to suggest conspecificity. There being no gametocytes of this organism in the MAPS smear, and the large size of its schizonts with abundant cytoplasm and merozoites 1.2–1.4 μm in diameter eliminating subgenus *Novyella*, the author would have tentatively assigned it to *Haemamoeba*, had not Garnham's figures 19 and 20 shown two smallish, elongate gametocytes. Pending more plentiful material, it is proposed to leave the identification at *Plasmodium* ***incertae sedis.***

Plasmodium (Giovannolaia) dissanaikei de Jong 1971

One of the best descriptions of an avian malaria parasite in recent years was Dr. Audrey de Jong's (1971) account of *P. dissanaikei* from a Sri Lankan host, the Rose-ringed Parakeet, *Psittacula krameri* (Scopoli) 1769 [WN 382.3]. This *Plasmodium* had been mentioned by Laird and Grewal (1968) as "an apparently new species of *vaughani*-like parasite with up to 10 and 12 small merozoites" from *Amaurornis phoenicurus* in Malaysia. Dr. de Jong resolved the matter, only erring in assigning her species to subgenus *Novyella*.

While 64% of her schizonts yielded only eight merozoites, others formed 9, 10 and 12. The upper limit was beyond that for all known species of *Novyella* except *P. nucleophilum*, but she nevertheless assigned *P. dissanaikei* to "the subgenus *Novyella* because it has schizonts with scanty cytoplasm and eight merozoites". Laird (1978) transferred this parasite to subgenus *Giovannolaia*, recognizing from de Jong's meticulous description and fine colour plate that *P. dissanaikei* schizonts cannot be said to have scanty cytoplasm by comparison with all known members of subgenus *Novyella*. He observed that "the resemblances among *P. dissanaikei, P. garnhami, P. durae* and *P. polare* are so close that there is no justification for retaining *P. dissanaikei* in *Novyella* while accepting the suitability of the others for placement within *Giovannolaia*".

According to de Jong (1971), merozoites of *P. dissanaikei* invade mature erythrocytes. Typical ring stages are rare. Once trophozoites have attained about 2–3 μm in diameter they tend to lie towards a pole of the host cell. Their cytoplasm then becomes visible "as small pseudopodial projections giving the parasite a fimbriated appearance" (de Jong 1971). Fine yellowish-brown granules of pigment appear, and developing schizonts become closely associated with the host-cell nucleus. Nuclear division begins when the schizont attains 4.5–5.0 μm, the chromatin masses usually moving "to the periphery giving the parasite a fan-shaped appearance". Maturing schizonts form 6–12 nuclei, 64% having 8, 25% having 6 and 3% having 12. From the earliest stages of schizogony, 1–6 circular refractile globules are scattered irregularly in the cytoplasm. Following segmentation dispersed merozoites often remain within the host cell, the nucleus of which may become slightly displaced. Developing gametocytes have a "tail-like" process. Mature ones are 13.2–14.4 μm long, extending the length of the host cell and "showing a slight tendency to curve round" its nucleus. Their medial border is very irregular, and they do not displace the erythrocyte nucleus, which "appears to be in strands or whorls extending more than half the length of the parasite". Clumped or diffuse pigment is plentiful.

The heaviest incidence of *P. dissanaikei* in MAPS slides was recorded from *Amaurornis phoenicurus* and *Trichastoma rostratum*. Twelve of the former and seven of the latter (Table 6.5) were parasitized by it. Of the 79 examples of *A. phoenicurus* sampled, 23 (29.1%) were malarious (Table 2.2). Seventeen (7%) of 242 *T. rostratum* were *Plasmodium*-positive too, one of them (from Rantau Panjang, Malaysia) actually exhibiting a triple infection of *P. dissanaikei, P. matutinum* and *P. elongatum*, besides also harbouring *Atoxoplasma* sp. The heaviest infections due to *P. dissanaikei* showed asynchronicity, the full range of asexual stages being represented in their smears.

Newly invaded merozoites were seen anywhere in the host-cell cytoplasm, but more than three were never present in the same corpuscle. Typical rings (1.5–2.0 μm diameter) were uncommon. They usually lay in the latero-polar region, but occasionally alongside the host-cell nucleus.

Table 6.5 Findings of ***Plasmodium (Giovannolaia) dissanaikei***

Host species[1]	Numbers recorded	Associated haematozoa[2]	Localities	Months
Dryocopus javensis	1	–	Palawan, Philippines	May
Loriculus galgulus	1	*H. handei*	Lowland Malaysia	May
Loriculus galgulus	1	*T, H. handei*	Lowland Malaysia	May
Trichoglossus haematodus	1	*H. handei*	Kuala Lumpur, Malaysia	May
Streptopelia chinensis	1	–	Palawan, Philippines	March
Amaurornis phoenicurus	1	–	Rantau Panjang, Malaysia	April
Amaurornis phoenicurus	1	*P.r.s.l.*	Rantau Panjang, Malaysia	April
Amaurornis phoenicurus	1	*P.v.*	Rantau Panjang, Malaysia	April
Amaurornis phoenicurus	1	–	Subang, Malaysia	February
Amaurornis phoenicurus	1	mf	Subang, Malaysia	June
Amaurornis phoenicurus	1	–	Subang, Malaysia	July
Amaurornis phoenicurus	1	*P.n.*	Subang, Malaysia	August
Amaurornis phoenicurus	1	*At*	Subang, Malaysia	September
Amaurornis phoenicurus	1	*At, P.v.*	Subang, Malaysia	October
Amaurornis phoenicurus	1	–	Subang, Malaysia	November
Amaurornis phoenicurus	1	–	Subang, Malaysia	November
Amaurornis phoenicurus	1	–	Subang, Malaysia	December
Porzana cinerea	1	–	Rantau Panjang, Malaysia	April
Rallina fasciata	1	*P.v.*	Luzon, Philippines	September
Ixobrychus sinensis	1	–	Dalton Pass, Luzon, Philippines	March
Dicrurus annectans	1	*P.v.*	Subang, Malaysia	October
Pycnonotus goiavier	1	*L, P.ci.*	Bang Phra, Cholburi, Thailand	October
Pycnonotus melanoleucos	1	*H, P.n.*	Sara Buri, Thailand	January
Trichastoma rostratum	2	–	Rantau Panjang, Malaysia	July, Dec.
Trichastoma rostratum	1	*P.r.s.l.*	Rantau Panjang, Malaysia	April
Trichastoma rostratum	1	*P.m.*	Rantau Panjang, Malaysia	July
Trichastoma rostratum	2	*At*	Rantau Panjang, Malaysia	June, July
Trichastoma rostratum	1	*P.m., P.e., At*	Rantau Panjang, Malaysia	March
Motacilla alba	1	*P.m.*	Rajasthan, India	January
Totals 13 host species and 31 individuals +ve *P. dissanaikei*				

[1] Taxonomic order as in Table 2.2.

[2] *Trypanosoma (T), Haemoproteus* (*H*, with species name where possible), *Leucocytozoon (L), Plasmodium* [*P. relictum* ***sensu lato*** *(P.r.s.l.); P. matutinum (P.m.); P. circumflexum (P.ci.); P. vaughani (P.v.); P. nucleophilum (P.n.); P. elongatum (P.e.)*], *Atoxoplasma (At)* and microfilariae (mf).

Some developing schizonts become tear-drop-shaped as the volume of chromatin increases, their pointed end increasingly filopodial and the overall length about 4.5 μm. Polar examples curve about the tip of the host-cell nucleus, usually touching it. Most growing schizonts have only one fine filopodium, snaking out like the 7.4 μm one arrowed in Figure 6.38. (This particular example has a second filopodium only slightly extruded on the right side of the schizont, and two others at its base.) The longest filopodium seen had emerged from a 9.5 × 3.5 μm schizont. It measured 12.5 μm, having five sinuosities and a tiny chromatin dot terminally. This dot recalled that for the far shorter "tail" reported from Haiba (1948) from some trophozoites of *P. rouxi*. de Jong's (1971) description of the "pseudopodial projections" of developing trophozoites of *P. dissanaikei* and the "tail-like" process of immature gametocytes reveal the presence of conspicuous filopodia in her material, as do her Figures 11–13. Incipient filopodia arrowed in the left-hand schizont of Figure 6.39 (the right ones of this parasite and the right-hand schizont having terminal chromatin knobs) correspond to de Jong's pseudopodial projections. A far longer filament (tip arrowed) from the right-hand schizont of Figure 6.39 has passed beneath the host-cell nucleus. Such remarkably long filopodia bear an intriguing resemblance to those of the saurian parasite, *Plasmodium (Carinamoeba) rhadinurum* Thompson and Huff 1944.

As schizonts mature and cytoplasm becomes less prominent, filopodia disappear. Mature hexanucleate schizonts are seen in Figures 6.40 and 6.41. Both are from the same slide, a joint infection with *P. (Novyella) nucleophilum* and *P. dissanaikei* in *Amaurornis phoenicurus*. The example of Figure 6.40, with its central pigment dot, is a presegmenter of *P. nucleophilum*. Figure 6.41 shows the same stage of *P. dissanaikei*, with its relatively much larger chromatin masses in fan configuration. Little cytoplasm is evident. A refringent granule is arrowed, and the nuclei are so crowded that their full number could only be distinguished under the microscope, with maximum light. Figure 6.42 shows the final stage of development of a *P. dissanaikei* schizont with ten uncondensed nuclei, resembling that of de Jong's figure 7. The arrow indicates a dense central clump of yellowish-brown pigment. A segmenter with eight condensed merozoites (1.2–1.3 μm diameter) is seen in Figure 6.43 (pigment arrowed), the host erythrocyte and its nucleus being entirely unaffected by the parasite's presence. de Jong's (1971) careful illustrations show nuclear displacement to be usually slight, as it was in the MAPS material. Only occasionally was there minor tilting of the host-cell nucleus, when large segmenters with 10 (Figure 6.44) or 12 (Figure 6.45) merozoites were involved.

The following range of merozoite counts from 100 mature schizonts/segmenters compares de Jong's results from *Psittacula krameri* in Sri Lanka with those from MAPS *Amaurornis phoenicurus* in Malaysia.

Table 6.6 Comparison of results: MAPS versus de Jong (1971)

No. of merozoites per schizont/segmenter	6	7	8	9	10	11	12
No. of schizonts/segmenters (de Jong)	25	0	64	3	5	0	3
No. of schizonts/segmenters (MAPS)	28	2	55	0	10	0	5

The gametocytes of this parasite seen in MAPS material agreed with their description by de Jong (1971) in being robust, deep-staining and not displacing the host-cell nucleus. Unhappily, the package of Zeiss Axiomat photographs portraying them was water-damaged in transit from Newfoundland to New Zealand, so they are not illustrated here.

The above morphological data identify the MAPS material from *Amaurornis phoenicurus* as *Plasmodium dissanaikei*. Examples from all other hosts listed in Table 6.5 were likewise fully comparable, as are their ecological preferences, with that of the type host. The Rose-ringed Parakeet, which extends eastward from Sri Lanka and India to lowland Myanmar and Hong Kong, and was at one time introduced to Malaysia where it may have died out (King and Dickinson 1975), is a bird of open woodland, savannah and farmland (Sibley and Monroe 1990). Interestingly, 61 examples of five species of *Psittacula* were sampled during MAPS, all of them proving negative for *Plasmodium.* However, three other parrots were found to harbour *P. dissanaikei* in lowland Malaysia, as were four other avian hosts there and seven more from elsewhere in the Asian Tropical Subregion from India to the Philippines (Table 6.5). All infections in the two commonest hosts, *Amaurornis phoenicurus* (12) and *Trichastoma rostratum* (7) were from lowland Malaysia. These species are both particularly identified with marshes in light forest and cultivation frequented elsewhere by *Psittacula krameri.* This is now revealed as just one of many hosts instead of *the* natural one (as the bird from which an avian malaria parasite is first described is so often styled). The other *P. dissanaikei* hosts of Table 6.5 are either primarily associated with natural marshlands, paddyfields or mangrove swamps, or likely to be present in such habitats; none of which support any of the five mosquito taxa from London laboratory colonies with which de Jong (1971) tried unsuccessfully to obtain sporogonic development of this parasite.

7

Plasmodium (Novyella)

Plasmodium (Novyella) vaughani Novy and MacNeal 1904

Plasmodium vaughani was described (although barely recognizably) by Novy and MacNeal from the American Robin, *Turdus [migratorius] migratorius* Linnaeus 1766 [WN 761], from Ann Arbor, Michigan, USA. With synonyms, it is the second most frequently reported avian *Plasmodium* to *P. (Haemamoeba) relictum* **s.l.**, and geographically it is almost as widely reported as the latter (Garnham 1966; Bennett, Whiteway and Woodworth-Lynas 1982; Bennett *et al.* 1992). It appears to have a low degree of synchronicity (Garnham 1966). Its synonyms still continue to cause confusion, the satisfactory resolution of which would require monographic treatment. In order of appearance, these synonyms are: *P. tenue* Laveran and Marullaz 1904; *P. tumbayaensis* Mazza and Fiora 1930; *P. hexamerium* Huff (1935); *P. oti* Wolfson (1936b); and *P. octamerium* Manwell (1968). In his competent redescription of *P. vaughani*, Manwell (1935a) sunk *tenue* and *tumbayensis* as synonyms. He later (1949) synonymized *oti* with *P. hexamerium*. Garnham (1966) retained the latter as a valid species, but Bennett, Whiteway and Woodworth-Lynas (1982) listed both it and *P. octamerium* as probable synonyms of *P. vaughani*. By then, though, Seed and Manwell (1977) were according full specific status to *P. hexamerium*, *P. octamerium* and a resurrected *P. tenue*. In their catalogue of subsaharan avian haematozoa, Bennett *et al.* (1992) recognized only *P. vaughani* and *P. octamerium*. Their use of the latter name was simply repeating the usage of Manwell and Rossi (1975) who had listed a number of records of Manwell's (1968) proposed species, and of Ashford *et al.* (1976) who followed on the work of Manwell and Rossi with African field studies.

All the above synonyms are regarded herein as *P. vaughani*, which may well have legitimate subspecies, such as ssp. *merulae* (Corradetti & Scanga 1972) and ssp. *tenue* (emend. Corradetti and Scanga 1973); but which will be referred to hereunder by its specific name without further elaboration.

Most of the infections in MAPS birds (Table 7.1) were chronic ones. In the heaviest, only about 1% of the red cells were parasitized. In the lightest, 2.5 h elapsed before the first *Plasmodium* was found. Multiple

Table 7.1 Findings of ***Plasmodium (Novyella) vaughani***

Host species[1] (individual positive records)	Associated haematozoa[2]	Localities	Months
Turnix suscitator	–	Kuala Lumpur, Malaysia	December
Turnix suscitator	*T*	Kuala Lumpur, Malaysia	October
Turnix suscitator	*P.p.*	Kuala Lumpur, Malaysia	December
Turnix suscitator	*P.p.*	Kuala Lumpur, Malaysia	April
Turnix suscitator	*P.r.*	Bayawan, Negros Oriental, Philippines	December
Phaenicophaeus javanicus	*H. centropi*	Bukit Besi, Malaysia	August
Prioniturus discurus	*H. handai*	Basay, Negros Oriental, Philippines	December
Prioniturus platenae	–	Palawan, Philippines	December
Glaucidium cuculoides	*H. syrnii, L*	Sakaerat, Pakthong Chai, Thailand	June
Chalcophaps indica	–	Sara Buri, Thailand	January
Chalcophaps indica	*P.r.* **s.l.**, *P.n.*	Sara Buri, Thailand	January
Treron curvirostra	*P.m.*	Kuala Lumpur, Malaysia	December
Amaurornis phoenicurus	*H. gallinulae*	Sabah, E. Malaysia	September
Amaurornis phoenicurus	*P.d.*	Rantau Panjang, Malaysia	April
Amaurornis phoenicurus	*P.r.*	Tarabanan, Palawan, Philippines	April
Amaurornis phoenicurus	*P.d., At*	Subang, Malaysia	October
Rallina eurizonoides	–	Luzon, Philippines	June
Rallina eurizonoides	*H. gallinulae, P.n.*	Dalton Pass, Luzon, Philippines	July
Rallina fasciata	*P.d.*	Dalton Pass, Luzon, Philippines	December
Pitta erythrogaster	–	Aborlan, Palawan, Philippines	August
Pitta erythrogaster	*H*	Mt Makiling, Luzon, Philippines	August
Pitta moluccensis	*H, P.r.*	Rantau Panjang, Malaysia	August
Lanius cristatus	*H. lanii, P.r.* **s.l.**	Ping-tung, Taiwan	September
Lanius cristatus	*H. lanii, P.m.*	Siaton, Negros, Philippines	January
Lanius cristatus	*H. lanii, P.m.*	Batangas, Calatagan, Luzon, Philippines	September
Oriolus chinensis	mf	Negros, Philippines	March
Oriolus chinensis	*H, P.ci.*, mf	Siaton, Negros Oriental, Philippines	November
Dicrurus annectans	*P.p.*	Subang, Malaysia	October
Dicrurus annectans	*P.d.*	Subang, Malaysia	October
Dicrurus balicassius	*H, L, P.p., At*	Basay, Negros Oriental, Philippines	December
Dicrurus hottentottus	*H, P.r.r., P.r.*	Central Thailand	January
Turdus cardis	–	Japan	February
Turdus cardis	*L*	Tsunoshima, Yamaguchi, Japan	April
Turdus chrysolaus	–	Luzon, Philippines	March
Turdus obscurus	*L*	Mt Brinchang, Malaysia	November
Turdus obscurus	*T, L, P.r.*	Mt Brinchang, Malaysia	September
Zoothera sibirica	*P.r.*	Mt Brinchang, Malaysia	November
Zoothera sibirica	*P.r.*	Mt Brinchang, Malaysia	December
Zoothera sibirica	*P.r.* **s.l.**, *P.r.*	Mt Brinchang, Malaysia	December
Copsychus malabaricus	*P.r.*	Kuala Lumpur, Malaysia	September
Copsychus malabaricus	*H. fallisi*, mf	Palawan, Philippines	May
Copsychus malabaricus	*At*, mf	Subang, Malaysia	September
Copsychus saularis	–	Rantau Panjang, Malaysia	August
Copsychus saularis	*H. fallisi*	Subang, Malaysia	October
Copsychus saularis	*P.r.* **s.l.**	Koh Kred, Pak Kred, Thailand	January

Table 7.1 (*cont.*)

Host species[1] (individual positive records)	Associated haematozoa[2]	Localities	Months
Copsychus saularis	*H. fallisi*, *P(H)* sp?, *P.r.*	Subang, Malaysia	June
Copsychus saularis	*P.r.*	Mt Brinchang, Malaysia	January
Luscinia cyane	*P.r.* **s.l.**, *P.r.*	Tsunoshima, Yamaguchi, Japan	May
Pycnonotus blanfordi	*H*	Koh Kred, Pak Kred, Thailand	August
Pycnonotus cafer	*P.r.*	Sakaerat, Pakthong Chai, Thailand	October
Pycnonotus cafer	*L*, *P.r.* **s.l.**	Bharatpur, Rajasthan, India	October
Pycnonotus goiavier	*P.r.*	Kuala Kangsar, Malaysia	October
Pycnonotus jocosus	*H. sanguinis*	Sunday Market, Bangkok, Thailand	June
Pycnonotus melanoleucos	*L*	Nakhon Ratchasima, Thailand	June
Pycnonotus melanoleucos	*P.ci.*	Sakaerat, Pakthong Chai, Thailand	June
Pycnonotus plumosus	*P.r.*	Iwahig, Palawan, Philippines	March
Pycnonotus sinensis	*L*	Hong Kong	December
Zosterops japonicus	*P.m.*, *P.n.*	Chiang Mai, Thailand	December
Acrocephalus orientalis	–	Shinhama, Ichikawa, Chiba, Japan	May
Locustella lanceolata	*H*, *P.r.* **s.l.**	Pasi, Oriental Mindoro, Philippines	September
Orthotomus sutorius	*H. wenyoni*	Bukit Besi, Malaysia	August
Alcippe poioicephala	–	Taiwan	September
Pomatorhinus hypoleucos	*L*, *P.r.*, *At*, mf	Mt Brinchang, Malaysia	February
Pomatorhinus schisticeps	mf	Taiwan	September
Stachyris poliocephala	–	Gombak, Malaysia	February
Stachyris poliocephala	*H*, mf	Gombak, Malaysia	January
Stachyris poliocephala	*P.r.*, mf	Kuala Lumpur, Malaysia	May
Stachyris poliocephala	*At*, mf	Gombak, Malaysia	February
Yuhina zantholeuca	*H. timalus?*, *P.r.*	Chanthaburi, Thailand	February
Yuhina zantholeuca	*H. timalus?*, *P.r.*	Chanthaburi, Thailand	February
Yuhina zantholeuca	*H. timalus?*, *P.r.*	Chanthaburi, Thailand	February
Galerida cristata	*H. alaudae*	Bandar Abbās, Iran	?
Dicaeum cruentatum	*T*, *P.r.* **s.l.**	Kuala Kangsar, Malaysia	October
Aethopyga shelleyi	–	Puerto Princessa, Palawan, Philippines	May
Emberiza rutila	*H. fringillae*	Chiang Mai, Thailand	December
Totals 44 host species and 75 individuals +ve *P. vaughani*			

[1] Taxonomic order as in Table 2.2.

[2] *Trypanosoma (T), Haemoproteus (H,* with species name where possible), *Leucocytozoon (L), Plasmodium [P. (Haemamoeba)* sp?, *P(H)* sp?; *P. relictum* ***sensu lato*** *(P.r.s.l.); P. relictum* ssp. *relictum (P.r.r.); P. matutinum (P.m.); P. circumflexum (P.ci.); P. polare (P.p.); P. dissanaikei (P.d.); P. rouxi (P.r.); P. nucleophilum (P.n.)]; Atoxoplasma* sp? *(At)* and microfilariae (mf).

invasions were infrequent. The diameter of newly invasive *P. vaughani* merozoites did not exceed 0.7 μm (see dispersed merozoites of a hexanucleate segmenter, still within the parasitized erythrocyte of Figure 6.15). Some early trophozoites were solid and amoeboid. Others were oval (as arrowed in Figure 7.1a), ring-form (Figure 7.1b) or somewhat pyriform, as illustrated by Manwell (1935a). Signet rings had the usual clear central zone. Figure 7.1a was from a mixed infection of *Haemoproteus gallinulae*,

P. vaughani and *P. nucleophilum*, the distinctly smaller size of the latter's rings being evident at the same magnification from Figures 7.2 and 7.3. As Figure 7.1b was from a mixed infection with an unidentified haemoproteid only, there was no question in this case of any confusion with another species of *Plasmodium*. Although Garnham stated that "No typical ring forms with a vacuole are produced" by *P. vaughani*, these had been illustrated in earlier Asian Tropical Subregion material (Laird and Lari 1958; Laird 1962).

Older trophozoites and developing schizonts had proportionately more cytoplasm than the equivalent stages of *P. rouxi* (pp. 74, 76). However, like other representatives of subgenus *Novyella*, they had substantially less cytoplasm than characterizes *Giovannolaia* and *Huffia*, and still less than in *Haemamoeba*. Towards the first chromatin division a blackish pigment granule is usually apparent. This is sometimes accompanied by a clear refringent granule, which tends to disappear as Giemsa stain fades. The quadrinucleate presegmenters of Figures 6.17 and 6.18, their vacuolated cytoplasm faded, each show a pigment dot at the tail of the merozoite fan. Two even tinier ones are barely visible near the upper and lower limits of the cytoplasm (Figure 6.18). The roughly triangular or cone shape of the developing merozoites is characteristic. Cruciform (St Andrew's Cross) presegmenters, a pigment dot central (Figure 7.4), are common. A hexanucleate segmenter of *P. vaughani*, its closely packed merozoites rounded up, is the left-hand example in the doubly occupied cell of Figure 7.5. Its quadrinucleate associate still has triangular and uncondensed chromatin masses, presumably resulting from a slightly later merozoite invasion of the host corpuscle. Displacement of the latter's nucleus is clearly a consequence of the pressure of two parasites from the same side. Figure 6.14a,b illustrate the smaller size of the merozoites resulting from hexanucleate segmentation, those from octonucleate segmentation being smaller still (Figure 6.16). Figure 6.15 shows the fully condensed merozoites resulting from segmentation of a relatively large hexanucleate schizont of *P. vaughani*.

Average overall dimensions for *P. vaughani* schizonts and their uncondensed nuclei are 4.5×2.1 μm and 1.0×0.7 μm, respectively. The *Novyella* with which their quadrinucleate schizonts is most likely to be confused is *P. rouxi*, schizonts and uncondensed nuclei of which have average measurements of 3.1×1.7 μm and 0.9×0.5 μm, respectively. Once the merozoites have condensed to their final spherical shape and begun to disperse, the diameter of those of *P. vaughani* averages 0.7 μm and those of *P. rouxi* about 0.5–0.6 μm. While these size differences between the two species appear trifling, reference to Figures 7.4 (*P. vaughani*) and 7.6b (*P. rouxi*) will show that they *can* be differentiated visually when the former's segmentation is quadrinucleate. However, as Garnham (1966) observed, this "needs an intimate knowledge of these parasites". Figure 7.7a, showing a quadrinucleate segmenter of *P. corradettii* n.sp., provides further evidence of the care that must be taken in distinguishing between species of subgenus *Novyella*. The size of its condensed merozoites is close to that of *P. vaughani* in Figure 7.4, only the central pigment dot of the latter differentiating it from *P. corradettii* n.sp. in the monochrome photomicrograph. Were

Figure 7.7a in colour, though, it would be seen that the central space between the merozoites was fully occupied by a patch of light golden pigment. The quadrangular or box-form schizonts of Figure 7.8a,b are each from a pure infection. The first, of *P. vaughani*, shows no pigment. In the second, of *P. corradettii* n.sp., a terminal mass of brownish-golden pigment is arrowed (see also pp. 85–86).

Parasitaemia was too low in most MAPS smears exhibiting *P. vaughani* for meaningful calculation of the relative incidence of four, six or eight merozoites in each of the 44 host species. The following count was obtained from 100 successive mature schizonts and segmenters in a random search of numerous slides without reference to host or locality: four (55%), six (31%), eight (14%).

An earlier count from Malaysia involving relatively heavy infections in two of the present hosts (*Phaenicophaeus javanicus* and *Dicaeum cruentatum*) gave quite similar results (Laird 1962): four (65%), six (26%), eight (9%).

It is generally accepted that the outline of the host red cell and the position of its nucleus are seldom more than slightly affected by the presence of the diminutive *P. vaughani*, except after relatively rare double invasions (e.g. Figure 7.5) or when a gametocyte causes lateral pressure as in Figures 7.9 and 7.10b. As Garnham (1966) states, the gametocytes do not curve about the poles of the host-cell nucleus to any great extent. Growing ones frequently exhibit "Little tags of cytoplasm" terminally (Figure 7.11) and macrogametocytes have the inner border "much crinkled" (Figure 7.9). Garnham draws attention to the variability in number of the black pigment granules of the sexual stages, ranging from two in the Italian strain of Corradetti *et al.* (1961) through 4–5 in material from the USA (Manwell 1935a) and 8–11 in a Malaysian strain (Laird 1962) up to 24 in his own Kenyan strains (Garnham 1966). Malaysian macrogametocytes ranged from 9.4 to 13.6 μm $\times$ 1.2 to 2.6 μm (av. 11.3 $\times$ 1.8 μm), that of Figure 7.9 measuring 10.8 $\times$ 2.7 μm.

Seventy-five MAPS birds of 44 host species (Table 7.1) were found positive for *P. vaughani* across the breadth of the Asian Tropical Subregion from Rajasthan, India, to the Philippines, Hong Kong and Taiwan, with extensions into the Eurasian-African Temperate Subregion — westward to Iran and eastward to Chiba, Japan. *Galerida cristata*, the Iranian host, occurs from Africa and Europe to the Korean Peninsula. A bird of open country and farmlands, it (the Crested Lark) has resident and migratory races. Gaud and Petitot (1945) recorded *P. vaughani* from the Crested Lark in Morocco. Mohammed (1958) reported the same association from Egypt on three separate occasions when numerous other passerines proved negative. A migratory race of *G. cristata* might therefore be one of many west-east migrants capable of dispersing *P. vaughani*; which has now been listed from this host in the Kiev area of the Ukraine, Georgia, Tadzhikistan and Kazakhstan by Glushchenko (1962; 1963), Burtikashvili (1971; 1978), Subkhonov (1972a) and Yakunin (1976), respectively. The parasite was identified from several birds in Japan by Kano (1950), and (as both *P. hexamerium* and *P. tenue*, with no mention of *P. vaughani!*) by Manwell, Allen and Kuntz (1976) from Taiwan.

Plasmodium (Novyella) rouxi Sergent, Sergent and Catanei 1928

The type host for the tiniest of the avian malaria parasites was neither the laboratory canary from which the original strain of *P. rouxi* was derived, nor *Passer hispaniolensis*, afterwards shown to be a natural host in Algeria. It was the invertebrate vector, *Culex pipiens* **s.l.**, wild-caught examples of which had been used to infect the canary — having already infected another canary with *P. (Haemamoeba) relictum*, a fortnight earlier (Garnham 1966).

The latter fact is of great interest, bearing in mind that of the 75 individual birds found positive for *P. rouxi* during MAPS, five were also parasitized by *P. relictum* **s.l.**; as well as six with *P. matutinum* (commonly confused with *P. relictum* in blood-smear surveys) and 20 with *P. vaughani*. This suggests a commonality of vectors (Table 7.2). Table 7.2 also lists precisely the same number of individual parasitized birds as did Table 7.1 for *P. vaughani*, and with almost as many host species (38 versus 44).

Like *P. vaughani*, *P. rouxi* has a low degree of synchronicity (Wolfson 1936a). Most of the infections of Table 7.2 were very light, the first parasite found not being recorded before 30 min and seldom before 2 h. Although more than one parasite was rarely found per host cell, three newly invaded merozoites were once seen in a polychromatophil. Otherwise, very few examples of double invasions (some proceeding to developing trophozoites and schizonts) were encountered in MAPS slides. This differs from earlier Malaysian experience, when 3% of invaded cells (mature erythrocytes) in an August smear from *Pycnonotus goiavier* (Kuala Kangsar, Perak) exhibited two parasites, "(trophozoite/trophozoite, schizont/schizont, schizont/segmenter)" (Laird 1962).

The diameter of the just-invaded merozoite was, like that of the fully condensed ones still intracellular following segmentation, about 0.5 μm as is supported by the meticulous drawings of Mohammed (1958). Signet-ring trophozoites are rare (Laird 1962). With growth, the important diagnostic stage first observed by Mohammed (1958) becomes apparent. This is the "bow-tie" schizont, in which one or two dot-like, brownish pigment granules and (sometimes) a refractive globule are located at the constricted "knot" between two elongate-triangular chromatin masses (figure 3 of Mohammed 1958; figures 8, 9 of Laird 1962; Figure 7.12 herein).

Both chromatin masses now divide again, but not necessarily synchronously (Figure 7.13). Such asynchronous behaviour also occurs, equally rarely, in *P. vaughani* (Figure 6.16, where the uppermost nuclear mass of an octonucleate fission has yet to divide). Just as outstanding a difference between the latter parasite and its close relation, as is their relative merozoite size, is the fact that in *P. rouxi* more than four merozoites *never* result (Figure 7.14). That figure showing the consequences of a rare (and in this case certainly synchronous) double invasion has the large refractive (or "vitreous") globule of each arrowed. Cruciform (Figure 7.7b) and quadrangular or "box form" (Figure 7.6a) segmenters

Table 7.2 Findings of ***Plasmodium (Novyella) rouxi***

Host species[1] (individual positive records)	Associated haematozoa[2]	Localities	Months
Turnix suscitator	*P.v.*	Bayawan, Negros Oriental, Philippines	December
Ninox philippensis	*H. syrnii, P.f.*	Basay, Negros Oriental, Philippines	November
Ninox scutulata	–	Pandan, Sarawak, E. Malaysia	December
Otus lempiji	*H. syrnii*	Chiang Mai, Thailand	January
Otus lempiji	*H. syrnii, P.p.*	Subang, Malaysia	June
Otus sunia	*H. syrnii, P.f.*	Sara Buri, Thailand	January
Otus sunia	*H. syrnii, P.n.*	Sara Buri, Thailand	January
Amaurornis phoenicurus	*P.p.*	Rantau Panjang, Malaysia	April
Amaurornis phoenicurus	*P.v.*	Tarabanan, Palawan, Philippines	April
Ixobrychus cinnamomeus	*H. mathislegeri*	Laguna de Bay, nr. Manila, Philippines	October
Pitta moluccensis	*At*	Malaysia	June
Pitta moluccensis	*H, P.v.*	Rantau Panjang, Malaysia	August
Chloropsis cyanopogon	*L*, mf	Bukit Besi, Malaysia	August
Lanius cristatus	*P.m.*	Aborlan, Palawan, Philippines	August
Dicrurus hottentottus	*H, P.r.r., P.v.*	Central Thailand	January
Turdus obscurus	–	Luzon, Philippines	November
Turdus obscurus	*L*, mf	Mt Brinchang, Malaysia	March
Turdus obscurus	*T, L, P.v.*	Mt Brinchang, Malaysia	September
Zoothera sibirica	–	Mt Brinchang, Malaysia	August
Zoothera sibirica	–	Mt Brinchang, Malaysia	March
Zoothera sibirica	–	Mt Brinchang, Malaysia	November
Zoothera sibirica	–	Mt Brinchang, Malaysia	March
Zoothera sibirica	*L*	Mt Brinchang, Malaysia	January
Zoothera sibirica	*P.v.*	Mt Brinchang, Malaysia	November
Zoothera sibirica	*P.v.*	Mt Brinchang, Malaysia	December
Zoothera sibirica	*P.r.s.l., P.v.*	Mt Brinchang, Malaysia	December
Copsychus malabaricus	–	Kuala Kangsar, Malaysia	October
Copsychus malabaricus	–	Chiang Mai, Thailand	October
Copsychus malabaricus	*H. fallisi*	Chiang Mai, Thailand	May
Copsychus malabaricus	*H. fallisi*	Ranong, Thailand	April
Copsychus malabaricus	*L*	Ranong, Thailand	April
Copsychus malabaricus	mf	Muar, Malaysia	June
Copsychus malabaricus	*P.v.*	Kuala Lumpur, Malaysia	September
Copsychus malabaricus	*T, H. fallisi*	Kuala Kangsar, Malaysia	October
Copsychus saularis	*P.m.*	Rantau Panjang, Malaysia	January
Copsychus saularis	*P.m.*	Rantau Panjang, Malaysia	May
Copsychus saularis	*P.m.*	Rantau Panjang, Malaysia	September
Copsychus saularis	*P.m., P.v.*	Mt Brinchang, Malaysia	January
Copsychus saularis	*H. fallisi, P.*sp?, P.v.	Subang, Malaysia	June
Luscinia cyane	–	Gombak, Malaysia	October
Luscinia cyane	*P.r.s.l.*	Subang, Malaysia	September
Luscinia cyane	*P.m., At*	Subang, Malaysia	November
Luscinia cyane	*P.r.s.l., P.v.*	Tsunoshima, Yamaguchi, Japan	May
Sturnus nigricollis	*Ae, H. pastoris*	Bang Phra, Cholburi, Thailand	February
Hypsipetes leucocephalus	*L*	Chiang Mai, Thailand	October
Ixos amaurotis	–	Tsunoshima, Yamaguchi, Japan	October
Ixos philippinus	–	Camp Lookout, Negros Oriental, Philippines	September

Table 7.2 (*cont.*)

Host species[1] (individual positive records)	Associated haematozoa[2]	Localities	Months
Pycnonotus blanfordi	*H. octocompsae*	Koh Kred, Pak Kred, Thailand	August
Pycnonotus cafer	*L*	Sakaerat, Pakthong Chai, Thailand	June
Pycnonotus cafer	*P.v.*	Sakaerat, Pakthong Chai, Thailand	October
Pycnonotus flavescens	*H. sanguinus, L*	Chiang Mai, Thailand	December
Pycnonotus goiavier	–	Kuala Kangsar, Malaysia	October
Pycnonotus goiavier	*H*	Lanao del Norte, Luzon, Philippines	May
Pycnonotus goiavier	*P.v.*	Kuala Kangsar, Malaysia	October
Pycnonotus leucogenys	*H*	Bandar Abbās, Iran	?
Pycnonotus melanicterus	*H*	Bangkok, Thailand	May
Pycnonotus melanoleucos	*H, P.r.***s.l.**	Sara Buri, Thailand	January
Pycnonotus plumosus	–	Palawan, Philippines	?
Pycnonotus plumosus	*P.v.*	Iwahig, Palawan, Philippines	March
Prinia flaviventris	*H. sylvae, P.r.***s.l.**	Northern Thailand	January
Heterophasia melanoleuca	*H. timalus*	Chiang Mai, Thailand	February
Minla strigula	*L*	Mt Brinchang, Malaysia	January
Minla strigula	*T, At*, mf	Mt Brinchang, Malaysia	March
Pomatorhinus hypoleucos	*L, P.v., At*, mf	Mt Brinchang, Malaysia	February
Pomatorhinus schisticeps	*P.n., At*	Chiang Mai, Thailand	October
Pteruthius flaviscapis	–	Mt Brinchang, Malaysia	October
Stachyris poliocephala	*P.v.*, mf	Kuala Lumpur, Malaysia	May
Trichastoma rostratum	–	Mt Brinchang, Malaysia	June
Trichastoma rostratum	–	Mt Brinchang, Malaysia	August
Trichastoma rostratum	–	Mt Brinchang, Malaysia	November
Trichastoma rostratum	*P.co.*	Rantau Panjang, Malaysia	September
Trichastoma rostratum	*P.p.*	Rantau Panjang, Malaysia	February
Yuhina zantholeuca	*H. timalus?, P.v.*	Chanthaburi, Thailand	February
Yuhina zantholeuca	*H. timalus?, P.v.*	Chanthaburi, Thailand	February
Yuhina zantholeuca	*H. timalus?, P.v.*	Chanthaburi, Thailand	February

Totals 38 host species and 75 individuals + ve *P. rouxi*

[1] Taxonomic order as in Table 2.2.

[2] *Aegyptianella (Ae), Trypanosoma (T), Haemoproteus (H,* with species name where possible), *Leucocytozoon (L), Plasmodium* [*P. relictum* **sensu lato** *(P.r.s.l.); P. relictum* ssp. *relictum (P.r.r.); P. matutinum (P.m.); P. fallax (P.f.); P. polare (P.p.); P. vaughani (P.v.); P. nucleophilum (P.n.); P. corradettii* n.sp. *(P.co)*], *Atoxoplasma* sp. *(At)* and microfilariae (mf).

of *P. rouxi* show no sign of cytoplasm, and even a tiny dot of pigment (Figure 7.15) is seldom present. This differentiates them from quadrinucleate examples of the same stages of both *P. vaughani* (deciding between the two can be difficult; see Gaud and Petitot 1945) and *P. corradettii* n.sp. Those of the latter when freshly stained display this species' uniquely large patch of brownish-gold pigment (Figure 7.7a) as well as having merozoites appreciably larger (Figure 7.6b; 0.7–0.9 μm) than those of *P. rouxi* (Figure 7.6a; 0.5–0.6 μm). Such a level of precision in measurement is of course likely to be illusory should this particular factor be the only basis for taxonomic differentiation; for individual size variation of merozoites within the species under comparison, and technological variables such as fixation and staining may alter the apparent size of such small bodies.

Studying some considerably heavier infections, with more abundant mature schizonts and segmenters than in the MAPS material, Laird (1962) noted from relatively freshly stained slides that the refractive body was present in about 75% of these stages from Malaysian birds; all but one of which represented species sampled during MAPS. Malaysian smears from the latter revealed an incidence of 55%, and Philippines ones, only 23%. The overall average for MAPS material was 32%. This structure's recognition in *P. rouxi*, as in *P. vaughani*, thus seems subject to a complex of variables, doubtless including strains too.

After leaving the host cell, merozoites of *P. (Novyella)* species are commonly ingested by phagocytes (Figures 7.16–7.18). The first two figures are from mixed infections, *P. rouxi* + *P. vaughani* and *P. rouxi* + *P. corradettii* n.sp. Figure 7.16 is from *Trichastoma rostratum*, and Figure 7.17 from *Zoothera sibirica*. Both illustrate a possible source of confusion with exoerythrocytic schizonts of *P. (Huffia) elongatum*. Figure 7.18, from the same *Z. sibirica* smear, shows a more advanced stage of phagocytosis.

Gametocytes of *P. rouxi* (Figures 7.10a, 7.19) are distinctly smaller than those of *P. vaughani* (Figure 7.10b and p. 73). Those of the former species range from 8.2 μm to 11.7 μm $\times$ 1.1 μm to 2.4 μm, averaging 9.9 $\times$ 1.7 μm (Laird 1962). Figures 7.10a and 7.19 show mature sexual stages of *P. rouxi*, the latter a microgametocyte (9.8 $\times$ 1.7 μm) and the former a macrogametocyte (10.6 $\times$ 2.1 μm). The macrogametocyte's stranded nucleus is appreciably larger than the microgametocyte's compact one. Brownish-black pigment is scanty in both.

Seventy-five MAPS birds of 38 host species harboured *P. rouxi*. They covered much the same Asian Tropical Subregion range, with extensions beyond to Iran and Japan, as did *P. vaughani*. Twenty individual birds of 15 host species and three orders (Turniciformes, 1; Gruiformes, 1; Passeriformes, 13) had mixed infections of both parasites. As Tables 6.5 and 7.1 show, most listings of both were from passeriforms although there was a scattering of records for each from non-passeriforms (with about twice as many of these from *P. vaughani*). This is much in accord with the global literature as reviewed by Bennett, Whiteway and Woodworth-Lynas (1982) and Bennett *et al.* (1992). The finding of *P. rouxi* on the Japanese breeding grounds of two birds that winter in the Asian Tropical Subregion (Table 7.2) pointed to the significance of migratory species in the dispersal of avian malaria parasites. One of these hosts, *Luscinia cyane* (the Siberian Blue Robin), was also harbouring *P. vaughani* and *P. relictum* **s.l.** Its early summer occurrence at Tsunoshima suggests the possibility of relapse due to migration stress, and it is noted that gametocytes of *P. rouxi* were present. Moreover, of three *P. rouxi*-positive *L. cyane* sampled in Malaysia (September, October, November), one was also parasitized by *P. relictum* **s.l.** and another by *P. matutinum* (Table 7.2). Especially "good" avian malaria hosts such as the Siberian Blue Robin could be of prime importance in the long-distance transfer of such plasmodia.

Plasmodium (Novyella) nucleophilum Manwell 1935

Manwell (1935a,b) described *P. nucleophilum* from *Dumetella carolinensis* (Linnaeus) 1766, the Grey Catbird [WN 704] from Syracuse, New York, USA. Garnham (1966) could still call it a rare parasite in reviewing the few additional records that had accumulated over the three decades since its discovery, mainly from the United States and Central and South America. There was also an unconfirmed report from the cosmopolitan *Passer domesticus* in Egypt (Haiba 1948) and others from Japan (Kano 1950) and Malaysia (Sandosham *et al.* 1965). The former was from the Narcissus Flycatcher. *Ficedula narcissina* breeds from Honshu north to Hokkaido, wintering in the Asian Tropical Subregion. There, none of 44 MAPS examples sampled yielded *Plasmodium*. However, one (of 16) from Japan proved positive for a malaria parasite that, while it could not be identified below the genus level, was certainly not *P. nucleophilum*. The latter is so distinct, and proved during MAPS to be so prevalent in the Asian Tropical Subregion, that the author sees no reason to doubt Kano's (1950) finding. The Malaysian mention, that Sandosham *et al.* had taken no further than recognizing their parasite's resemblance to *P. nucleophilum*, was duly identified as such from a slide sent to Manwell (1966) from Sandosham. The latter's host was *Aplonis panayensis*, the gregarious Asian Glossy Starling, common throughout the Asian Tropical Subregion, and often closely associated with humans. MAPS material revealed the same association in Palawan, Philippines (McClure *et al.* 1978; and see p. 83), among 30 species of birds harbouring *P. nucleophilum* (Table 7.3).

In *P. nucleophilum*, with its 24 h cycle, "Parasitaemia is usually low and synchronicity of development is slight" (Garnham 1966). As Manwell and Voter (1939) pointed out, mature erythrocytes were usually the cells invaded, polychromatophils only exceptionally so. However, whether invasive or phagocytosed, merozoites were frequently present. The diameter of such merozoites seldom exceeded that of condensed and newly dispersed ones still within the host corpuscle, about 0.7 μm (Figure 7.20 upper group). The youngest stage recognized as a trophozoite is arrowed at the far left of Figure 7.21. Its diameter is 1.0 μm, and under the microscope a faint smudge of cytoplasm was barely evident below the chromatic spot. A minute vacuole appears with continuing growth (Figure 7.21, lower left curved arrow). Until this stage there has been no contact with the nucleus of the host cell. Mini-rings from a diameter of about 1.4 μm now move to the host-cell nucleus (Figures 7.2, 7.3), usually towards or at one pole as shown. Double invasions of the same erythrocyte are commonplace. These involve either simultaneous entry by two merozoites, or sequential entry leading to one parasite still showing no post-merozoite development, while the other has grown to the stage seen in Figures 7.2 and 7.3 (or perhaps to the twinned schizonts of Figure 7.22).

From now onwards *P. nucleophilum* clings tightly to the host-cell nucleus (Figure 7.21, central arrow), although the bond may be broken by the pressure of smearing. This is shown in Figure 7.23a, where the schizont having completed its first nuclear division bears a superficial

Table 7.3 Findings of ***Plasmodium (Novyella) nucleophilum***

Host species[1] (individual positive records)	Associated haematozoa[2]	Localities	Months
Gallus gallus	*Ae, P.r.**s.l.***	Palawan, Philippines	May
Eudynamys scolopacea	*P.r.**s.l.***	Palawan, Philippines	May
Otus lempiji	*H. noctuae, P.f.*, mf	Chiang Mai, Thailand	October
Otus sunia	*H. syrnii, P.n.*	Sara Buri, Thailand	January
Chalcophaps indica	*T, P.m., P.co.*	Tarabanan, Palawan, Philippines	May
Chalcophaps indica	*P.r.**s.l.**, P.v.*	Sara Buri, Thailand	January
Phapitreron leucotis	*T*	Lanas del Norte, Luzon, Philippines	March
Streptopelia chinensis	*T, P.co.*	Siaton, Negros Oriental, Philippines	February
Amaurornis phoenicurus	*P.d.*	Subang, Malaysia	August
Rallina eurizonoides	*H*	Dalton Pass, Luzon, Philippines	July
Sarcogyps calvus	*T*	Siaton, Negros, Philippines	December
Ixobrychus cinnamomeus	*H*	Laguna de Bay, nr Manila, Philippines	October
Pachycephala grisola	*P.e.*	Mt Brinchang, Malaysia	February
Oriolus chinensis	–	Siaton, Negros, Philippines	November
Zoothera cinerea	–	Dalton Pass, Luzon, Philippines	January
Acridotheres tristis	–	Kutch, India	March
Aplonis panayensis	*Ae, L, P.r.r.*, mf	Puerto Princessa, Palawan, Philippines	May
Sarcops calvus	*T, H. pastoris*	Siaton, Negros, Philippines	November
Sturnus nigricollis	*H. pastoris, P.ci.*	Bang Phra, Cholburi, Thailand	December
Pycnonotus melanicterus	*H. sanguinis*	Chiang Mai, Thailand	September
Pycnonotus melanoleucos	*H, P.d.*	Sara Buri, Thailand	January
Zosterops japonicus	*P.m., P.v.*	Chiang Mai, Thailand	December
Acrocephalus aedon	*P.r.**s.l.***	Chiang Mai, Thailand	January
Locustella fasciolata	*At*	Camp Lookout, Valencia, Luzon, Philippines	September
Pomatorhinus schisticeps	*P.r., At*	Chiang Mai, Thailand	October
Anthreptes malacensis	–	Tarabanan, Palawan, Philippines	May
Nectarinia jugularis	*P.m., P.co.*	Tarabanan, Palawan, Philippines	May
Ploceus manyar	*P.m.*	Sunday Market, Bangkok, Thailand	March
Ploceus philippinus	*Ae, H. quelea*	Bang Phra, Cholburi, Thailand	August
Ploceus philippinus	*P.r.**s.l.***	Kutch, India	March
Lonchura punctulata	–	Koh Kred, Pak Kred, Thailand	August
Emberiza aureola	–	Chinchup-Myun, South Korea	August
Totals 30 host species and 32 individuals +ve *P. nucelophilum*			

[1] Taxonomic order as in Table 2.2.

[2] *Aegyptianella (Ae), Trypanosoma (T), Haemoproteus (H,* with species name where possible*), Leucocytozoon (L), Plasmodium* [*P. relictum* ***sensu lato*** *(P.r.**s.l.**); P. relictum* ssp. *relictum (P.r.r.); P. matutinum (P.m.); P. circumflexum (P.ci.); P. fallax (P.f.); P. dissanaikei (P.d.); P. vaughani (P.v.); P. rouxi (P.r.); P. nucleophilum (P.n.); P. corradettii (P.co.); P. elongatum (P.e.)*] and *Atoxoplasma (At).*

resemblance to the "bow-tie" stage of *P. rouxi*. There is a tiny pigment dot between the parasite's medial vacuole and the arrowed cleft where it has been pulled away from the erythrocyte nucleus. The attachment face is often at a "shoulder" of that nucleus, as shown in the cases of the multinucleate schizonts of Figures 7.3, 7.23b and 7.24. The second of these schizonts has not been artificially displaced, but is voluntarily moving away to undergo segmentation. All four schizonts have bright little vacuoles in the cytoplasm, which is much more abundant than in *P. rouxi*. The pigment cannot be distinguished except in Figure 7.25, which exhibits a single brownish-black clump at lower left. A hexanucleate schizont (possibly destined for a final division into 12) with a similar dot of pigment is illustrated in Figure 6.40. It is so positioned for easy comparison with the equivalent stage of *P. (Giovannolaia) dissanaikei* of Figure 6.41, both being from the same *Amaurornis phoenicurus* slide.

The tangential interface so often evident between a latero-polar *P. nucleophilum* schizont and the "shoulder" of the host-cell nucleus (along the side of which it has spread) is arrowed in Figure 7.24. A definite preference for this attachment site is apparent from the fact that a count of 134 successive *P. nucleophilum* schizonts from a random selection across all MAPS hosts revealed 111 (83%) to occupy the "shoulder" position. This is a useful although previously overlooked recognition feature for the parasite. It shows to particular advantage as segmenting schizonts relinquish their hold (Figure 7.26a) when vacuolated cytoplasm becomes less evident as condensation into merozoites begins. It is inapparent from early schematic illustrations, but the colour illustrations in Garnham (1966) — taken from an American blood film supplied by Manwell — make the point. His plate LVI, figures 18 and 21 show the initial "shoulder" attachment. This becomes less clear in some of the larger schizonts as they grow along the host-cell nucleus, for example, the octonucleate ones of Figure 7.27 herein and Garnham's plate LVI, figure 19. The tangential nature of the "shoulder" attachment plane is often so straight as to suggest lysis of the nucleus by the parasite. That this is not so, though, is apparent from the frequency of such a plane towards an end of the nucleus of perfectly normal avian red cells and others where there is no parasite contact with the nucleus (e.g. Garnham's plate LVI, figure 16).

There is occasionally minor displacement and slight tilting of the host-cell nucleus by the larger schizonts (Figure 7.27), especially in double invasions where the parasites are located at obliquely opposite interfaces. More merozoites may be formed by *P. nucleophilum* than by any other known *Novyella*. A count of 73 segmenters randomly selected across all MAPS hosts gave the following incidences of merozoite numbers (Table 7.4):

Table 7.4 Incidences of merozoite numbers across MAPS hosts

No. of merozoites	4	5	6	7	8	9	10	11	12
No. of segmenters	19	6	31	0	10	3	2	0	2
Percentage of segmenters	26	8	42	0	14	4	3	0	3

Odd numbers are relatively rare, with 8% at five and 4% at nine. A presegmenter in process of forming nine merozoites is seen in Figure 7.28, still clamped to the host-cell nucleus and its pigment dot arrowed. The usual number is 4–9, with most mature schizonts/segmenters quadri- or hexanucleate. However, Lucena (1939) reported a range of 5–12 in his Brazilian strain. An example of the uppermost level (Garnham 1966, plate LVI, figure 22) was closely paralleled by a presegmenter with condensing merozoites, newly separated from its host-cell nucleus, in a Malaysian slide from *Amaurornis phoenicurus* (Table 7.3). One more MAPS *P. nucleophilum* slide (from *Aplonis panayensis*, Palawan, Philippines) yielded a 12-nucleate segmenter. It also had another with ten merozoites, as did a *Pycnonotus melanoleucos* from Sara Buri, Thailand (Table 7.3). There was no chance of confusion with double invasions in any of these three birds. However, Figure 7.26b from a Philippines *Streptopelia chinensis* shows two adjacent hexanucleate schizonts of *P. nucleophilum*, the arrow indicating the line of separation between them, that superficially resemble a *Giovannolaia* schizont as well as a 12-nucleate example of the parasite under discussion.

A double association of this kind can be still more misleading following the dispersal of both sets of condensed merozoites. Thanks to their being at slightly different stages of development, the two octonucleate sets of Figure 7.20 are easily distinguishable, but this would obviously not have been the case had the smear been made very shortly afterwards. Finally, the merozoites of what was presumably the segmentation of a hexanucleate schizont, are seen (perhaps due to pressure engendered in smearing) in the act of leaving the host cell in Figure 7.29. It should be added that the diameters of the condensed merozoites of *P. nucleophilum* average about 0.7–0.8 μm, or a shade more than those of *P. vaughani* (about 0.7 μm) and distinctly more than for *P. rouxi* (about 0.5–0.6 μm). Figure 7.30 (upper centre) shows two schizonts at very different stages of development in *Aplonis panayensis*.

Triple invasions of red cells by *P. nucleophilum* are rare. That seen in Figure 7.31 at upper centre shows a quinquenucleate schizont and a lower-left quadrinucleate one, with a later-invading merozoite at right. Figure 7.32 illustrates double occupancy of the same *Sturnus nigricollis* erythrocyte by a hexanucleate schizont of *P. nucleophilum* (curved arrow) and a *Haemoproteus pastoris* gametocyte (broad arrows). Gametocytes of the former typically adhere to the host-cell nucleus. Somewhat shorter than those of other species of *Novyella* (Garnham 1966), few were found in MAPS slides. Those of Figures 7.33 and 7.34 typically clamp to the host-cell nucleus, and their length approximates to the lower limit for *P. rouxi* (p. 77). The first illustrates a 7.7 × 2.1 μm microgametocyte; the second, an 8.5 × 3.1 μm macrogametocyte. The mature microgametocyte centrally above the scale-bar in Figure 7.35 measures 11.8 × 2.4 μm. It and the younger stage of Figure 7.33 exhibit clumped pigment and much resemble figure 26, plate LVI of Garnham (1966). All three gametocytes are broad enough to have caused minor lateral displacement of the host-cell nucleus. The first two are quite smoothly margined, as is often the case (Manwell 1966), but the microgametocyte of Figure 7.35 displays the irregular outline referred to by Sandosham *et al.* (1965).

Northeast of the Asian Tropical Subregion, Kano's (1950) record of this parasite from *Ficedula narcissina* in Japan is now augmented by the discovery of *P. nucleophilum* in *Emberiza aureola* from South Korea (Table 7.3). Like *F. narcissina*, this fringillid (which winters from India through Southeast Asia to the Philippines but breeds across the southern Eurasian-African Temperate Subregion) might well serve as a transport host for *P. nucleophilum* to and from the Asian Tropical Subregion. Furthermore, while there are no previous published reports of *P. nucleophilum* from the western approaches to the latter Subregion, MAPS blood smears include two positives from Kutch, in westernmost India. The hosts are the ubiquitous *Acridotheres tristis* and *Ploceus philippinus*.

Plasmodium (Novyella) juxtanucleare Versiani and Gomes 1941 (?)

Plasmodium juxtanucleare, the second malaria parasite of the Domestic Fowl, was described from Mias Gerais, Brazil. A year before, Africa, Dy and Soriano (1940) had reported plasmodia that Garnham (1966) believed "may" have been the same parasite, and therefore its first record from the Asian Tropical Subregion, in "a large number of medium-aged native Philippine chickens". Their plasmodia proved lethal to young native and white leghorn chicks on injection. They suggested the likelihood of it being *P. (Haemamoeba) gallinaceum*, and stated that the latter's describer, Brumpt, concurred on being shown the Philippines parasite. However, the authors' careful figures show the typical *P. juxtanucleare* association with the host-cell nucleus, and also "a few plasmodia which probably belong to another species". The latter were probably *P. (Giovannolaia) circumflexum*. The first certain report of the former parasite from the western side of the MAPS area was from Japan, where Ishiguro (1957a,b) believed that he had discovered an undescribed species and named it *P. japonicum*. Akiba (1959) recognized Ishiguro's error, and synonymized the latter's species with *P. juxtanucleare*; the earliest certain finding of which from the Asian Tropical Subregion was that of Dhanapala (1962) from Domestic Fowls in Sri Lanka, where Dissanaike (1963) provisionally identified this parasite from one of eight Ceylon Junglefowls, *Gallus [gallus] lafayettii* Lesson 1831.

Bennett *et al.* (1963) extended the distribution of *P. juxtanucleare* to Malaysia, finding it in Domestic Fowls at Kuala Lumpur and in a nearby coastal mangrove swamp, from which sporozoites from a naturally infected mosquito vector were injected into a chick and permitted elucidation of the full life cycle. The latter revealed the unique pedunculated oocyst of this species, which otherwise closely resembles *P. nucleophilum*. The chief differences in the blood stages are that the gametocytes of *P. juxtanucleare* are of round to oval shape and some 3.8–5.0 μm in length, appreciably smaller and far less elongate than those of *P. nucleophilum*; and that while the relationship of trophozoites and schizonts with the host-cell nucleus is the same in both species, no more than five (and usually four) merozoites are formed in the former species. At least, these were the figures derived from Domestic Fowl infections by South American and other earlier workers. Manuel, Tongson and Balediata (1969) confirmed the presence of *P. juxtanucleare* in Domestic Fowls in the Philippines, and Manuel and Dulay (1970) achieved experimental infections in Domestic Turkeys, *Meleagris gallopavo* Linnaeus 1758 [WN 310], there too. Meanwhile Manwell (1966) had reported what he believed to be *P. juxtanucleare* from 5 of 26 *Bambusicola thoracica* (Temminck 1815), the Chinese Bamboo Partridge [WN 2151], from Taiwan. From his description and illustrations there is nothing to differentiate his parasite from *P. nucleophilum*, aside from the fact that he found no more than four merozoites per segmenter. For in low parasitaemias, that is often the case in infections due to the latter species, and Manwell admitted that he found relatively few segmenters.

Nevertheless, Manwell (1966) was convinced that he had discovered a natural phasianid host of *P. juxtanucleare*, which Mohan and Manwell (1969) afterwards listed from an African bird of the same family, *Francolinus* sp. collected in Tanzania — despite the fact that single segmenters formed as many as eight merozoites. Earlé *et al.* (1991) have more recently recorded the species from *Francolinus [africanus] africanus* Greywing Francolin [WN 6093] in South Africa's Eastern Cape Province, giving the merozoite range as 3–9. Only two of their 21 infected birds had stages other than trophozoites present, making one wonder how 19 of the positives could possibly be differentiated from *P. nucleophilum*, while the photomicrographs from one of the two heavy infections showed decidedly more host-cell nuclear displacement and distortion than is typical for *P. juxtanucleare*. Dr. F. W. Huchzermeyer, one of Dr. Earlé's co-authors, was good enough to send the author of this book a heavily parasitized slide from *F. africanus*. This proved to contain both macro- and microgametocytes, which were neither mentioned nor illustrated in the above paper — and the author must concede that both sexual stages were completely in accord with the published accounts of those of *P. juxtanucleare*. However, there were also indications of a second species of subgenus *Novyella* being present, notably numerous bright-vacuoled signet-ring trophozoites. These, like that seen at the lower-left figure 4 of Earlé *et al.* (1991) do not occur in *P. juxtanucleare*, although they are plentiful in, for example, *P. vaughani* (Figure 7.1b), *P. nucleophilum* (Figure 7.2) and (especially) *P. corradettii* n.sp. (Figure 7.36). *P. corradettii* n.sp. also illustrates host-cell nuclear consequences of parasitism, not unlike those of the Earlé *et al.* Figure 4.

Unfortunately, no Domestic Fowls were sought by MAPS. However, as indicated in Chapter 5 (p. 39), 1 of 17 Red Junglefowls sampled near Puerto Princessa, Palawan, Philippines, was parasitized by a species of subgenus *Novyella* in addition to *P. relictum* **s.l.** and *Aegyptianella* sp. This (Figures 7.31, 7.37) was identified as *P. (N) nucleophilum* (Table 7.3), its invasive merozoites, trophozoites and quadrinucleate schizonts being inseparable from those of this parasite (compare Figure 7.30 from *Aplonis panayensis*, smeared on the same day in the same locality). In the absence of any round to oval gametocytes an identification of *P. juxtanucleare* would have been inadmissible.

It is generally assumed that *P. juxtanucleare* is confined to Phasianidae (Earlé *et al.* 1991), with all but a handful of reports being from the Domestic Fowl. The Domestic Fowl has been regarded as the sole host of *P. gallinaceum* except for a very few records from varieties of the wild Red Junglefowl in India, Sri Lanka and Malaysia. Therefore, it might have been tempting to so identify both parasites of the present Red Junglefowl from Palawan, simply on grounds of host occurrence, had it not been for the coincident occurrence of *P. nucleophilum* and *P. relictum* ssp. *relictum* in an *Aplonis panayensis* from the same habitat. For neither the *Haemamoeba* nor the *Novyella* of the Red Junglefowl showed any morphological differentiation from the Asian Glossy Starling plasmodia. The *Aegyptianella* from both hosts, which was morphologically identical to *A. pullorum*, may or may not have been this species, too.

Plasmodium (Novyella) corradettii n.sp.

Type host and date:	*Pitta brachyura* (10 August 1962)
Type locality:	Rantau Panjang, Malaysia
Hapantotype slide:	Deposited in the Department of Invertebrate Zoology, National Museum of Natural History, Smithsonian Institution, Washington, DC, USA: USNM: #47911
Parahapantotype slides:	From *Trichastoma rostratum* (Rantau Panjang, 6 September 1960) and *Nectarinia jugularis* (Tarabanan, Palawan, Philippines, 13 May 1962): registration numbers 1997:4:30:1 and 1997:4:30:2, respectively. Deposited in the Natural History Museum, London, UK, with the Garnham collection of malaria parasites and other Haemosporidia.
Other hosts:	*Chalcophaps indica* (Tarabanan, 13 May 1962) and *Streptopelia chinensis* (Siaton, Negros Oriental, Philippines, 17 February 1965)
Associated haematozoa:	See Table 7.5

The type locality was an extensive area of mangrove swamps at Rantau Panjang on Malaysia's west coast. *P. brachyura*, the Indian Pitta, and *T. rostratum*, the White-chested Babbler, are well known from this habitat, as is the Olive-backed Sunbird, *N. jugularis*. The other hosts, both doves, ranging from thick forest to adjacent road edges and cultivations, commonly encounter the mangrove habitat, too.

Plasmodium (Novyella) corradettii n.sp. — This fits the subgeneric criteria (see pp. 23–25). It is named in memory of a friend and distinguished malariologist, the late Prof. Augusto Corradetti, formerly

Table 7.5 Findings of ***Plasmodium (Novyella) corradettii n.sp.***

Host species[1] (individual positive records)	Associated haematozoa[2]	Localities	Months
Chalcophaps indica	*T, P.m., P.n.*	Tarabanan, Palawan, Philippines	May
Streptopelia chinensis	*T, P.n.*	Siaton, Negros Oriental, Philippines	February
Pitta brachyura	–	Rantau Panjang, Malaysia	August
Trichastoma rostratum	*P.r.*	Rantau Panjang, Malaysia	September
Nectarinia jugularis	*P.m., P.n.*	Tarabanan, Palawan, Philippines	May
Totals 5 host species and 5 individuals +ve *P. corradettii* n.sp.			

[1] Taxonomic order as in Table 2.2.

[2] *Trypanosoma (T), Plasmodium* [*P. matutinum (P.m.); P. rouxi (P.r.); P. nucleophilum (P.n.)*].

Direttore del Istituto Superiore di Sanita, Rome. It particularly honours his many contributions to avian malariology.

Trophozoites — These (Figure 7.38, right example, and Figure 7.36, two examples) form sturdy "signet rings", about 0.9–1.2. μm in diameter. Large for *Novyella*, their peripheral cytoplasm is often conspicuous (Figure 7.36, right example) until the prominent chromatin has spread around the periphery prior to the first nuclear division. The central clear zone may appear whitish in a freshly stained smear. There are frequent double invasions of mature erythrocytes, and sometimes triple ones. These invasions range from synchronous to decidedly asynchronous. In the latter case, as seen in the central example of Figure 7.36, there may be such an interval between merozoite invasions that two entirely different life-history stages are associated, a mature macrogametocyte and a signet-ring trophozoite.

Trophozoites commonly lie at or towards a host-cell pole. Others, as in the upper-right sector of Figure 7.36, occur laterally to the host-cell nucleus, but without touching it.

Schizonts — At their first formation, round to oval binucleate schizonts have a deep-staining chromatin mass at either extremity. Such early schizonts measure about 1.8×1.4 μm, their cytoplasm diminishing or disappearing entirely in those destined to form four merozoites only. The organism then becomes a pair of chromatin masses with an adjacent large disc of brownish-golden pigment (arrowed) as seen in Figure 7.38, lower-left. Such "dumb-bell' schizonts are the equivalent of the "bow-tie" ones of *P. rouxi* (Figure 7.12). They now undergo a second division, to form quadrinucleate schizonts; the separate nuclei of which may adopt a tightly cruciform configuration (Figure 7.6b), in which pigment is occasionally inapparent (especially in monochrome photomicrographs), occasioning possible confusion with the same stages of *P. vaughani* (Figure 7.8a) and the smaller *P. rouxi* (Figure 7.6a). Sometimes, too, the developing merozoites are so closely jammed that no free space separates them. As in other species of *Novyella*, fan-, box- and rosette-shaped segmenters may result. Perfect examples of the last-mentioned are seen in

Figures 7.39 (at left of erythrocyte immediately above scale line, the other two parasites in that cell being developing schizonts of *P. (N.) nucleophilum*) and 7.40 (pure infection in *Pitta brachyura*, the uppermost paler patch in the accompanying schizont being brownish-golden pigment). The fan-shaped schizonts can become virtually linear as in Figure 7.41 (showing initially pyriform division products) and Figure 3.1 (in which the merozoites are fully condensed and spherical).

The apparently quadrinucleate schizont (possibly destined for a hexanucleate one) of Figure 7.42 has the distinctive pigment patch of *P. corradettii* n.sp. (arrowed). An even larger such patch is arrowed in the hexanucleate segmenter of Figure 7.43, the parasite's extrusion intact from the host cell presumably having happened during smearing. Figures 7.44 and 7.45 show the characteristic brownish-yellow, virtually discoidal pigment patch well. Arrowed in both instances, it is two to three times the bulk of the condensing merozoites, and is centrally positioned in the irregular rosette of Figure 7.44. In Figures 7.42, 7.44 and 7.45, marked displacement of the host-cell nucleus is obvious, and the cell membrane appears to be in a delicate state (note partly extruded nucleus of the parasitized corpuscle of Figure 7.45). Later still, as the fully condensed and spherical merozoites begin to disperse (Figures 7.46, 7.47), with the previously conspicuous pigment disc fading or altogether disappearing, the host-cell membrane becomes fimbriated (arrows). Proneness of such cells to damage during smearing might account for the prevalence of extra-corpuscular segmenters and still-associated merozoites in some slides of *P. corradettii* n.sp? A fan-shaped quadrinucleate segmenter (top) and two cruciform ones, their merozoites rounded but not yet dispersed, are seen in Figure 3.1. The result of a simultaneous triple invasion of the host cell, it would be easy to confuse this with a 12-merozoite segmenter of a *Giovannolaia*. Figure 3.1, though, is from the only pure infection of *P. corradettii* found (Table 7.5), and the arrows show the separations between the three segmenters — note that the uppermost merozoite of the bottom example is precisely superimposed on the lowermost one of the middle example.

One hundred randomly selected maturing schizonts and segmenters from all five hosts were the basis for merozoite counts, 48% proving quadrinucleate, 38% hexanucleate and 14% octonucleate. The diameter of fully condensed merozoites was about 0.7–0.9 μm.

Gametocytes — Staining unusually deeply with Giemsa, these are fusiform to slightly crescentic or bean-shaped. Their outline is smooth. Both sexes exhibit a few bright vacuoles, an approximately central nucleus, and polar cytoplasm that is so densely stained as to recall the terminal caps of some haemogregarines (Figure 7.36). Pigment is scanty, consisting of small, blackish granules (Figure 7.48, top-right). The latter figure shows lateral displacement of the host-cell nucleus by a microgametocyte of *P. corradettii* n.sp. Macrogametocytes (Figure 7.36, an asynchronous double invasion of an erythrocyte exhibiting nuclear displacement and tapering towards the uppermost pole) range from 6.2 to 7.6 μm in length and 3.2 to 3.7 μm in breadth. In an erythrocyte from the Palawan Emerald Dove, a synchronous double invasion had led to the presence of two maturing gametocytes, one of each sex. Their host cell and its nucleus were both almost circular.

Discussion — The peripheral blood stages of *P. corradettii* n.sp. meet all morphological criteria for *Novyella*. Of the five earlier "good" species, *P. nucleophilum* and *P. juxtanucleare* are eliminated from comparison by reason of the tight adherence of their developing trophozoites and schizonts to the host-cell nucleus. *P. rouxi* is excluded on grounds of its appreciably smaller size, distinctive "bow-tie" binucleate schizonts and its fragile little gametocytes. While *P. vaughani* shares with *P. corradettii* n.sp. the occurrence of quadri-, hexa- and octonucleate mature schizonts/segmenters in a similarly descending order of incidence, three features rule it out of contention with the latter. First, its trophozoites and merozoites are smaller. Second, its gametocytes are *very* different. Third, and most importantly, the black pigment dots of *P. vaughani* schizonts are trivial by comparison with the relatively huge brownish-golden discs of *P. corradettii* n.sp.

The only avian malaria gametocytes comparable with those of the latter are found in *P. (N.) bertii* (Gabaldon and Ulloa 1981). They are smooth-margined in both, with similar staining characteristics, those of the latter (Venezuelan) species being somewhat the longer but not so stubby as in *P. corradettii*. A particular resemblance between them, though, is the tendency of their polar gametocytes to adopt the tangential position of Figures 7.36 and 7.49; and figure 24 of Gabaldon and Ulloa (1981). But despite these resemblances, *P. bertii*, like *P. rouxi*, never forms more than four merozoites; by comparison with four, six or eight in *P. corradettii* n.sp. And its pigment is slight when compared with the very large brownish-golden discs of the latter. Moreover, the marked displacement of the host-cell nucleus and/or fimbriation of the erythrocyte membrane, is unique to *P. corradettii* n.sp. with respect not only to *P. bertii* but to all other known representatives of subgenus *Novyella*.

P. corradettii n.sp. is thus proposed as a very distinct avian malaria parasite of subgenus *Novyella*, on grounds of its unique schizont pigment, the other morphological details named above, and its adverse effects upon both the nucleus and the cell membrane of the parasitized corpuscle.

8

Plasmodium (Huffia)

Plasmodium (Huffia) elongatum Huff 1930

The subgenus *Huffia*, with only two species, differs from all other avian malaria parasites in that its schizogony may occur in primitive blood-forming cells. Its type species, *P. elongatum*, was described by Huff (1930) not from the strain isolated by Dr. J. H. Boyd from *Passer domestics* in Georgia, USA, some 6 years earlier, but from one discovered by Dr. E. Hartman in Baltimore, Maryland, USA, in 1926, in a captive canary. This was in joint infection with *P. relictum*, and Dr. C. G. Huff duly isolated a pure strain from material supplied by Hartman, later in the same year. The type host for *P. elongatum* Huff (1930) is therefore *Serinus canarius* Linnaeus 1758, the Island Canary [WN 533.1] (previously the Common Canary or simply, Canary). Since used widely in experimentation, this parasite seems more prevalent than elsewhere in natural hosts in the USA.

In Garnham's (1966) list of natural hosts for *P. elongatum* from the Americas, Africa, Europe and Asia, he included several Philippines birds sampled some 35 years previously by Dr. Paul F. Russell. However, the latter had only claimed two of these, wild-caught (*Excalfactoria lineata*) = *Coturnix chinensis* and *Turnix (fasciata)* = *T. suscitator*, as probably carrying a Luzon strain of *P. elongatum*. Russell's (1932a) drawing of a gametocyte of *P. elongatum* could just as well pass for *P. vaughani*, *P. rouxi* or *P. polare*, all three of which were identified from MAPS *T. suscitator*; five examples of which harboured *P. vaughani*, two of them (from Malaysia) carrying *P. polare* as well, and one (from the Philippines) doubly infected with *P. rouxi*. Additionally, two Blue-breasted Quails (from the Philippines) and two Barred Buttonquails (from Malaysia) had very light infections with malaria parasites that could not be identified beyond the genus (Table 3.1). Both hosts yielded other plasmodia, too (Table 2.2 shows that in total 197 examples of *C. chinensis* and 141 of *T. suscitator* were studied). None of these slides exhibited *P. elongatum*, nor did any from the many other MAPS samples from the Philippines.

There are no other previous references to *P. elongatum* from the Asian Tropical Subregion, and only two from subsaharan Africa (Bennett *et al.* 1992). A few old records mentioned by Garnham from

North Africa stand in need of confirmation, notably those of Haiba (1948) from Egyptian *Passer domesticus*. Mohammed (1958) thoroughly investigated this host in Egypt and, while not encountering *P. elongatum*, found 58 of 176 House Sparrows to be parasitized by *P. rouxi*. Garnham (1966) had noted records of the former parasite from the eastern sector of the Eurasian-African Temperate Subregion concerning fringillids and muscicapids wintering in Japan from Korea, and within a decade or so of his book's publication, these were supplemented by reports from that Subregion's central sector. These related to two species of doves in Kazakhstan (Yakunin 1976; Yakunin and Zhazyltaev 1977) and the same two passerines from which Haiba had listed *P. elongatum* from Egypt but this time, from Tadzhikistan (Subkhonov 1972a). Surprisingly, although these authors on Kazakhstan avian malaria, also Zhazyltaev (1977), were very productive of new host and distribution records for *P. vaughani*, they made no mention of *P. rouxi* which was equally abundant with the former in MAPS material. It is easy to confuse these species, particularly *P. rouxi* with *P. elongatum*, the more so when phagocytosed merozoites are abundant in the smear (Figures 7.16–7.18; Laird 1953; 1962). Garnham's (1966) comment that from examination of a single blood film, "often only a tentative conclusion as to the identity of the parasite can be reached" is as applicable to much of the published work based on blood-smear surveys as to future research.

Only three MAPS birds, all from Malaysia, harboured *P. elongatum*. They were a White-chested Babbler, *Trichastoma rostratum* (Rantau Panjang, Selangor coast, 8 March 1960); a Mangrove Whistler, *Pachycephala grisola* (Mt Brinchang, Cameron Highlands, 10 February 1959); and a White-breasted Waterhen, *Amaurornis phoenicurus* (Rantau Panjang, 4 February 1960). The first also harboured *P. matutinum*, *P. dissanaikei* and *Atoxoplasma* sp.; the second, *P. nucleophilum*; and the third was a pure infection, and the most informative of these preparations. Sketches made from the pure infection after receipt in Geneva in 1965, showed merozoite invasions of both erythroblasts and late polychromatophilic erythrocytes. The few signet-ring trophozoites seen were located towards an end of the host cell. The largest measured 1.7 μm in diameter. No developing schizonts were found, and mature ones and segmenters were rare. Polar in location, they had usually displaced the host-cell nucleus towards the opposite pole, sometimes with tilting. Occasionally, though, nuclear displacement was scarcely evident. There was sometimes a single clump of blackish pigment at the point of junction of separating merozoites in a fan-shaped configuration, as illustrated in plate 2, figure 18 of Huff (1930). When the (usually half dozen) very long merozoites were in an irregular mass, the segmenter had a strange striated appearance (a peculiarity to which Dr. Clay Huff drew the author's attention on a visit near Washington, DC in 1950). In such cases the clumped pigment was central. Prior to condensation the merozoites, quite unlike any other avian malaria ones, measured about 5.5×1.2 μm. On dispersal within the red cell their dimensions became slightly less, their curved, elongate form being "quite reminiscent of *Toxoplasma gondii*" as Garnham (1966) observed.

Gametocytes were elongate, and of the "thin emaciated aspect" described by the latter author. As he stated, too, their inner margin was "usually irregular or digitated". This is shown in Figures 8.1 and 8.2, from the White-chested Babbler. Unusually narrow in proportion to their length, these gametocytes were separated from the host-cell nucleus by a decided gap. Otherwise, though, they had much in common with the *P. rouxi* gametocyte of Figure 7.10a. They measured about 11.6–1.9 μm to 12.6–1.7 μm, the convex margin being appressed to the host-cell membrane exactly as in Garnham's (1966) plate LVIII, figures 7 and 8. The parasitized corpuscle of Figure 8.1 measures 12.5 × 6.5 μm, while the average-sized, uninfected one at far-left centre is only 11.0 × 5.8 μm. This is again much in accord with the latter author's data, as is the paleness of the cytoplasm.

Turning to the exoerythrocytic stages of *P. elongatum*, trophozoites and schizonts were present in the *Amaurornis phoenicurus* smear in both small and large lymphocytes, and schizonts and segmenters were seen in monocytes. Figure 8.3 shows an immature schizont in either a normoblast or a thrombocyte, from the *Pachycephala grisola* slide. The ease of confusing such a stage of *P. elongatum* with phagocytosed merozoites of some species of *Novyella*, in this instance *P. nucleophilum*, is evident from comparison of this photomicrograph with Figures 7.17 and 7.18.

9

General discussion

Controversy over the validity of many of the nearly 80 species and subspecies of *Plasmodium* that have been described from birds (Bennett, Whiteway and Woodworth-Lynas 1982) will persist until much more is known of such matters as the morphological variability of the individual parasites in different hosts, both vertebrate and invertebrate. Most of the taxa that have been proposed are known only from stained avian blood films, and in so comprehensive a field survey as the present one, concomitant experimentation is usually impracticable.

Thus six species of bird plasmodia had been claimed to occur in Hawaii (where local transmission could not have occurred before the first establishment of mosquitoes, which took place as recently as 1826 (refs in Laird and van Riper 1981), prior to a project centred on the island of Hawaii itself in the late 1970s. By then several other potential vectors had reinforced the earliest one, the well-known transmitter of avian malarias, *Culex quinquefasciatus* Say, 1823. This project followed Warner's (1968) assertion that resultant mortalities were threatening the survival of non-immune birds endemic to Hawaii. It revealed the presence of only a single *Plasmodium, P. (Haemamoeba) relictum* ssp. *capistranoae*, extremely heavy infections of which yielded highly atypical parasites in some hosts (Laird and van Riper 1981). The type host and locality for this subspecies are *Coturnix chinensis* and Luzon, Philippines (Russell 1932b; and p. 33). Blue-breasted Quails, the bird in question, were imported into Hawaii as potential game in 1910, but failed to survive (Berger 1972). As reiterated by van Riper, Atkinson and Seed (1994), ssp. *capistranoae* "easily can be mistaken for different parasites when it develops in different hosts".

Besides this kind of obstacle to the certain identification of avian malaria parasites from peripheral blood films alone, especially when the number of examples for a particular host and locality is very limited, faulty fixation and staining are often attributable to field circumstances and can compound the problem. So, too, can the manner of representation of the various life-history stages of *Plasmodium* spp. in the publications that must be consulted for purposes of comparison with positive slides under microscopic examination. Relevant sketches differ widely in their quality, and the attractiveness of Giemsa staining can make painted versions impressive but misleading. Thus numerous colour illustrations in Garnham's (1966) book were made by a skilled artist from published monochrome drawings, in which connection the author can cite personal experience. For Garnham's figures 1–8 of plate LVI were painted from stippled camera-lucida drawings in Laird (1962), and critical comparison with the originals will reveal that accuracy has been diminished by artistry. To take but two examples, the delicate early ring-form trophozoite of *P. (N.) vaughani* in figure 23 of the latter has been transmuted to an aggressively heavy signet-ring in figure 1 of the former; while the whitish refractive globule of the same parasite's quadrinucleate schizont in figure 29 of the latter has become an inadmissibly highlighted blue ball in figure 4 of the former. Only photomicrography can solve the problem, and with today's rapidly increasing ISO ratings and improving colour saturation of colour films, these are destined to outdo monochromes as used herein. Unhappily, though, the fading of colour fiches of a pictorial guide to avian haematozoa made 22 years ago (Greiner *et al.* 1975) suggests that this approach to the ideal solution was premature.

The prime example of laboratory experimentation with living avian malaria parasites was of course the first elucidation of the complete sporogonic development of a *Plasmodium* (presumably *P. relictum* **s.l.**) in a mosquito now believed to have been *Culex quinquefasciatus*. The work of Ronald Ross (1898) was undertaken in the Asian Tropical Subregion in India. The parasitized birds on which the mosquitoes were fed were House Sparrows and larks, the former a particularly frequent host of *P. relictum* **s.l.** Four decades later the same Subregion was involved in another such episode concerning avian malaria, although not actually demonstrated to be so until now. For Coggeshall (1938) sampled the blood of (ex-Borneo) Crestless Firebacks at the New York Zoological Park, or Bronx Zoo, New York, USA, describing *P. (Giovannolaia) lophurae* from them and establishing a laboratory strain to which ducks soon proved highly susceptible and which later became adapted "almost completely to mice", providing "apparently the only example of the passage of a malaria parasite from one class of vertebrate to another" (Garnham 1966). When the latter work appeared, the possibility of this species having been acquired by the Crestless Firebacks from some local bird in New York was still entertained. The claims of Ogaki (1949) to have found *P. (G.) lophurae* in Malaysia were long since questioned as is indicated in Chapter 6 (p. 63), where more recent listings from numerous unlikely hosts in Kazakhstan are equally discounted. Mention of the species' occurrence in a solitary MAPS example of *Lophura erythropthalma* from Subang, Malaysia, was made by McClure *et al.* (1978), but without the morphological data now presented. A generation of malariologists had referred to Hewitt's (1940) plate VII for their visual impression of *P. (G.) lophurae*, in the stippled drawings based upon Coggeshall's (1938) illustrations in his original description. However, although the single laboratory strain survived, its ability to produce normal sexual forms had ceased long before the appearance of Garnham's (1966) book. The macrogametocyte of Figure 6.37 will be seen to accord very closely with its equivalent in Hewitt's (1940) plate VII, but rather less well with the work of Garnham's artist in his figure 13, plate LIII, adapted from Hewitt (1942).

Turning to the number of widely recognized species of avian malaria parasites, Hewitt (1940) listed 12 as "those which are almost universally accepted" in his table 3; which also included 19 others as synonyms, unconfirmed or controversial. His short-listed species were, as alphabetically presented: *P. cathemerium, P. circumflexum, P. elongatum, P. gallinaceum, P. hexamerium, P. lophurae, P. nucleophilum, P. oti, P. polare, P. relictum, P. rouxi* and *P. vaughani*. Nine of these were included among the certain MAPS species, the exceptions being *P. hexamerium* and *P. oti* (both now generally synonymized with *P. vaughani*) and *P. gallinaceum* (which while originally described from the Asian Tropical Subregion, has as its type host the Domestic Fowl, which was excluded from the MAPS mandate). Strangely, two of Hewitt's controversial species resurfaced in the "Key to Species Identification" closely following his table 3. One of these was *P. fallax* (with nine MAPS records from four avian hosts). The other was *P. paddae*, now synonymized with *P. relictum* **s.l.**

Garnham (1966) raised the total of acceptable species of *Plasmodium* of birds to 23. He added four subspecies, too, all of *P. relictum* — ssp. *capistranoae*, *spheniscidae*, *lutzi* and *subpraecox*. His additional valid species included *P. matutinum* (originally described by Huff (1937) as a subspecies of *P. relictum*) and *P. fallax*, *P. giovannolai* (post-dating Hewitt (1940) and a MAPS "possible", Chapter 5) and *P. juxtanucleare* (also post-dating Hewitt (1940) and like *P. gallinaceum* known from the Asian Tropical Subregion but, for the same reason as the latter, excluded from MAPS). To these Garnham added three species known only from very limited Asian Tropical Subregion material, *P. (Giovannolaia) anasum* and *P. (G.) formosanum* from Taiwan and *P. (Haemamoeba) griffithsi* from Myanmar. Only the host of the first was represented in the MAPS material, and that by just two slides, both negative. Garnham's valid list was further augmented by six little-known species of *Plasmodium*, only reported from Africa (4) and South America (2); plus the otherwise discredited *P. hexamerium*. His *P. relictum* ssp. *capistranoae* (regarded simply as a synonym of *P. relictum* by Hewitt (1940)) is added to the author's present list of valid taxa. So is Garnham's *P. relictum* ssp. *subpraecox*, since raised to specific status (Chapter 5, pp. 34–36). On the basis of Garnham (1966) the MAPS list, incorporating hereunder the subgenera of Corradetti, Garnham and Laird (1963a), stands at:

> ***P. (H.) relictum, P. (H.) relictum*** *ssp.* ***capistranoae, P. (H.) subpraecox*** *(suspected, but discarded as unlikely),* ***P. (H.) cathemerium*** *(possible identification),* ***P. (H.) matutinum, P. (H.) giovannolai*** *(possible identification),* ***P. (G.) fallax, P. (G.) circumflexum., P. (G.) polare, P. (G.) lophurae, P. (N.) vaughani, P. (N.) rouxi, P. (N.) nucleophilum*** *and* ***P. (H.) elongatum.***

The next important global register of avian malaria parasites was that of Bennett, Whiteway and Woodworth-Lynas (1982), which expanded the overall list to 70 species and five subspecies (of which 31 species were declared to be valid). All the above MAPS identifications were among the latter group. So were *P. gallinaceum, P. juxtanucleare* and nine of Garnham's (1966) ten other acceptable species. However, Bennett, Whiteway and Woodworth-Lynas (1982) rightly rejected

Garnham's continuing acceptance of *P. hexamerium*, favouring synonymizing it with *P. vaughani*. Two Asian Tropical Subregion species described since the latter's book appeared, *P. hegneri* Manwell and Kuntz (1966) from Taiwan and *P. dissanaikei* (Chapter 6, p. 63), were now added to the valid list (the type host of the former was represented in the MAPS collections by 123 blood slides, only two of which were from Taiwan — all were negative for *Plasmodium*). van Riper, Atkinson and Seed (1994) accept the Bennett, Whiteway and Woodworth-Lynas (1982) decisions on the current substantive list, adding only *P. bertii*. This very distinctive tropical American newcomer (p. 87) was described by Gabaldon and Ulloa (1981) some months before publication of the former authors' host-parasite catalogue of the avian haematozoa.

The final MAPS list thus stands at the indented block of 10 species, with the nominotypical subspecies and ssp. *capistranoae* of *P. (H.) relictum*, on p. 95; plus *P. (G.) dissanaikei* and *P. (N.) corradettii* n.sp. Except for the two Domestic Fowl parasites, *P. (H.) gallinaceum* and *P. (N.) juxtanucleare* (well known from and presumably evolved in the Asian Tropical Subregion and perhaps also in more northerly parts of China, but beyond the MAPS mandate), this list comprises all widely recognized species now known from our Subregion. It excludes four others recognized as valid by Bennett, Whiteway and Woodworth-Lynas (1982) and van Riper, Atkinson and Seed (1994) that were described on rather slim evidence from Taiwan — *P. (G.) anasum, P. (G.) hegneri* and *P. (G.) formosanum* — and Myanmar — *P. (H.) griffithsi*. The status of five more species ranges from "possible" to "unlikely" (p. xvii).

The overall percentages for all MAPS birds parasitized by *Plasmodium* spp. and the malarial index for *Plasmodium*-positive species only, were much as in earlier extensive surveys of large zones with highly diversified habitats and avian and culicine mosquito faunas — approximately 1% and 2%, respectively. As Table 2.2 shows, these incidences applied to most of the individual bird hosts. However, they were at variance with the suggestion of van Riper, Atkinson and Seed (1994) that good examples of taxonomic groups appearing to be infected commonly are Fringillidae, Emberizinae and Sturnidae. Thus of the 918 Fringillidae/Emberizinae of five species listed in Table 2.2, only six (0.65%) harboured *Plasmodium*; while for 995 Sturnidae of eight species the equivalent figures were 23% and 2.31%. Now the most numerous of the Sturnidae was *Aplonis panayensis*, the Asian Glossy Starling, only two (0.8%) of 259 of which were malarious; yet one of these, the example from Puerto Princessa, Palawan, Philippines, sampled on the same occasion as a Red Junglefowl (pp. 39 and 83), yielded one of the only two quintuple infections of the entire MAPS operation — *P. (N.) nucleophilum*, *P. (H.) relictum* ssp. *relictum*, *Leucocytozoon* sp., *Aegyptianella* (aff. *pullorum?*) and microfilariae. In the other quintuple infection, the subject of which was one (14.4%) of seven Large Scimitar-Babblers (*Pomatorhinus hypoleucos*), the parasites identified were *P. (N.) vaughani, P. (N.) rouxi*, *Leucocytozoon* sp., *Atoxoplasma* sp. and microfilariae (Table 7.1).

The Large Scimitar-Babbler belongs to the Sylviidae/Sylviinae/Timaliini, the Babblers, 1866 individuals of which, representing 14 species, were sampled. Just 39 birds (0.02%) of these *Plasmodium*-

harbouring species were malarious. But 17 or 7.2% of 242 examples of *Trichastoma rostratum*, the White-chested Babbler, harboured three species of *Plasmodium, P. (H.) matutinum, P. (G.) dissanaikei* and *P. (Huffia) elongatum*, besides microfilariae.

Again, of the 47 species of Rallidae mentioned as having been examined worldwide for haematozoa in Bennett, Whiteway and Woodworth-Lynas (1982), only nine (four of these being MAPS birds) harboured *Plasmodium*. But one of these marshland dwellers, the White-breasted Waterhen, *Amaurornis phoenicurus* (which is notably peridomestic; Whistler 1949) showed 23 positives (Table 2.2), amounting to 29.11% of the 79 examined from various locations. Twelve of these yielded *P. (G.) dissanaikei*, with three other species involved in double infections.

It is ventured that this and much other such information to be gleaned from the tables herein (but that would require a dauntingly large monograph to do justice to) suggests that it is by no means necessarily the family relationships of malarious birds that determine their incidence of infection, but the ecological circumstances within which they exist. The birds with particularly heavy mixed burdens of haematozoa instanced above, were all sampled in peridomestic environments, where in addition to a nearby wide range of natural larval mosquito habitats, there was a considerable diversity of artificial such habitats for such well-known vectors of avian malarias as *Culex quinquefasciatus* and *Aedes aegypti*. Such facts emerging from the MAPS data invite speculation on the likely evolution of both malaria parasites of that most peridomestic of all birds, the Domestic Fowl, within its native Asian Tropical Subregion and during the period of rather less than 5000 years since its domestication began.

Several of the Subregion's flourishing universities are ideally located as bases for the necessary investigations, and for others (notably studies of the role of migratory birds in the dispersal of avian species of *Plasmodium*) admirably suited to rewarding collaboration with researchers of the African-Eurasian Subregion, Australia and New Zealand. Contemporary awareness of the threat posed to many avian species through habitat depletion due to rainforest destruction and other such obvious factors as accidental and deliberate introductions of predators, has yet to be matched in this vast area of the globe by purposeful evaluation of bird morbidity and mortality due to malarial disease. It is high time that it were, and that sector of the MAPS fieldwork discussed here could serve as the necessary launching platform.

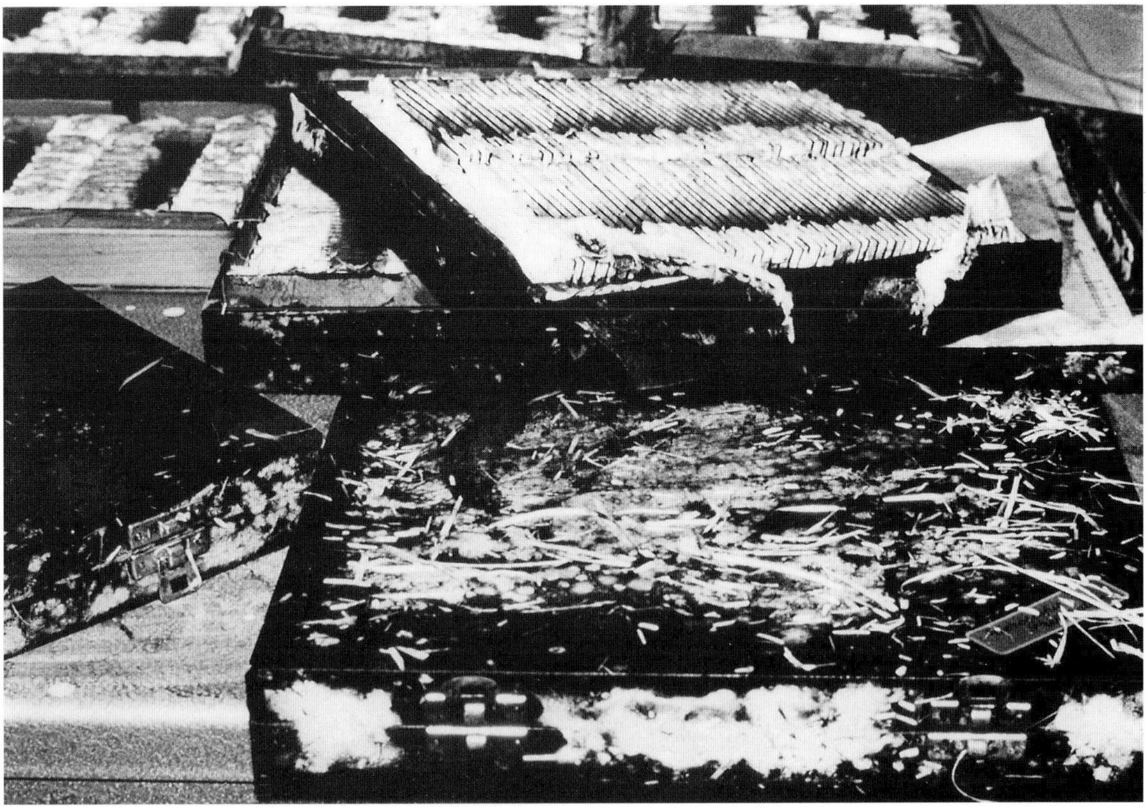

Figure 2.1 Damp slides with damaged labels shown, during unpacking from mouldy boxes in sodden packaging, following 1962 sea transportation from Malaysia.

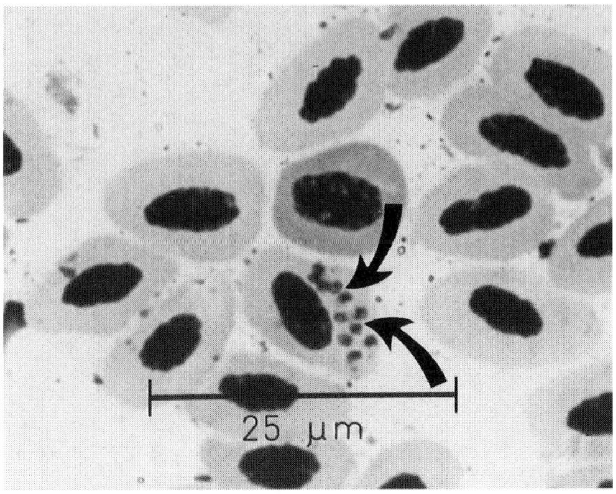

Figure 3.1 Not an elongate schizont of a member of the subgenus *Giovannolaia*, but three segmenters of *P. (Novyella) corradettii* (divisions between them arrowed), pure infection ex *Pitta brachyura*; Rantau Panjang, Malaysia, 10 August 1962.

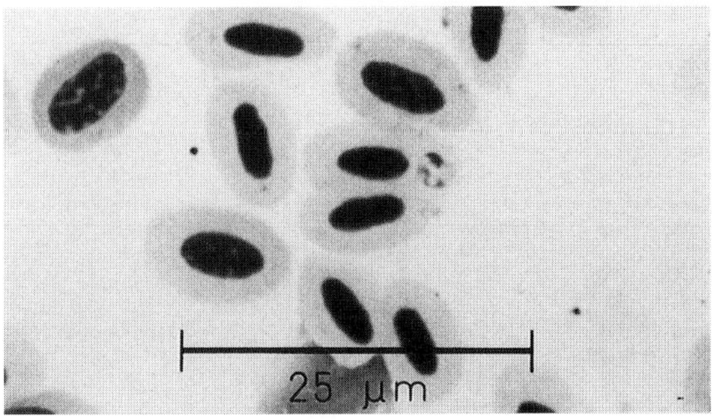

Figure 3.2 *Plasmodium* sp? ex *Trichastoma rostratum*; Rantau Panjang, Malaysia, 2 February 1961.

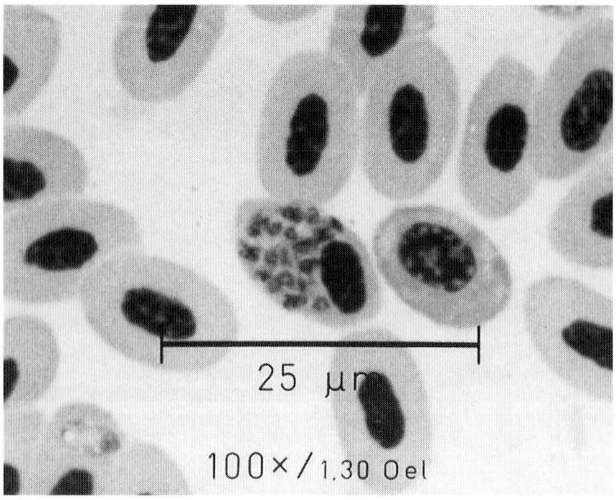

Figure 5.1 *Plasmodium (Haemamoeba) relictum* ssp. *relictum*, 16-nucleate schizont ex *Otus lempiji*; Nakhon Ratchasima, Thailand, 18 September 1967.

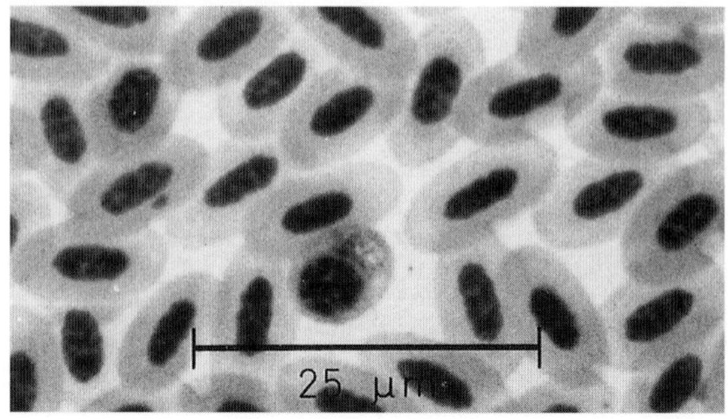

Figure 5.2 *P. (H.) relictum* ssp. *capistranoae* ex *Coturnix chinensis*, late trophozoite in erythroblast; Dalton Pass, Luzon, Philippines, 1 February 1965.

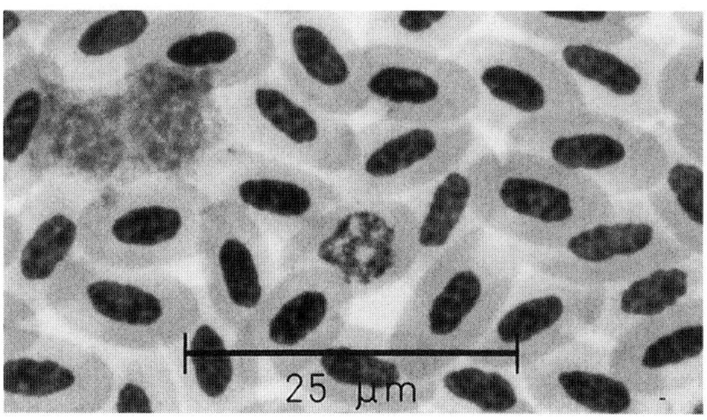

Figure 5.3 Same species and slide as Figure 5.2. Schizont in enucleated eythrocyte.

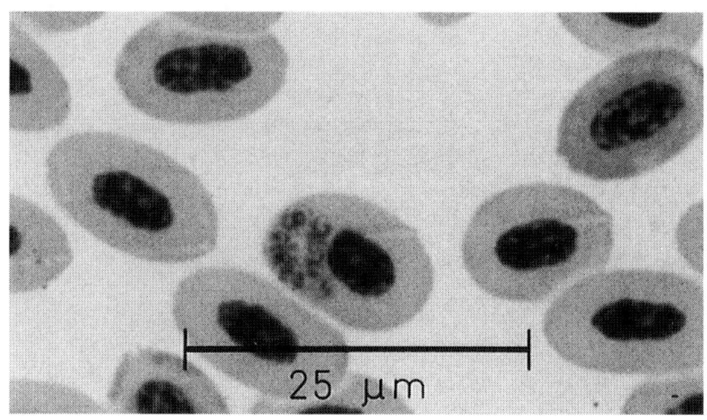

Figure 5.4 Schizont of *P. (Giovannolaia) fallax* (as a *P. (H.) subpraecox* look-alike) ex *Otus lempiji*; Nakhon Ratchasima, Thailand, 18 September 1967.

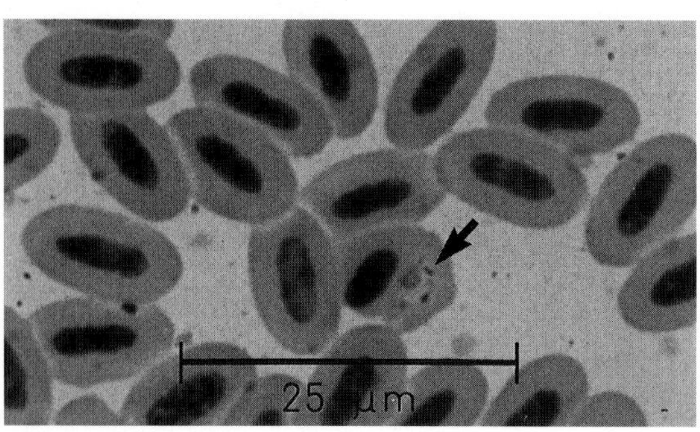

Figure 5.5 Early microgametocyte of *P. (H.) relictum s.l.*, resembling *P. (H.) cathemerium* (rod-shaped pigment granule arrowed), ex *Lonchura malacca*; Camarines Norte, Luzon, Philippines, 27 April 1965.

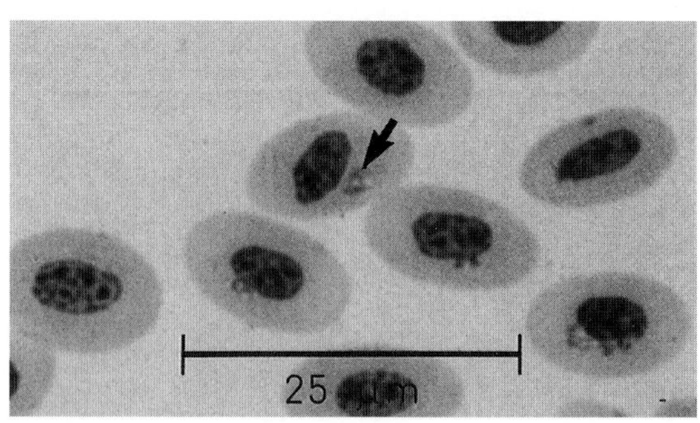

Figure 5.6 *P. (H.) relictum* ssp. *relictum*, ex Red Junglefowl (joint infection with *P. (N) nucleophilum*), early schizont arrowed; Puerto Princessa, Palawan, Philippines, 24 May 1962.

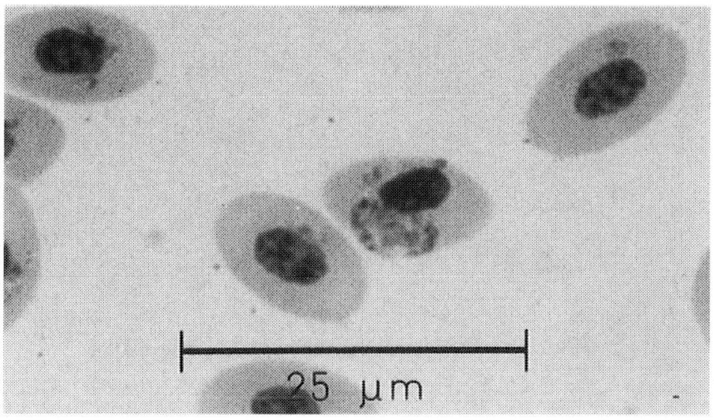

Figure 5.7 Same parasite and slide as Figure 5.6, developing schizont with 14 merozoites.

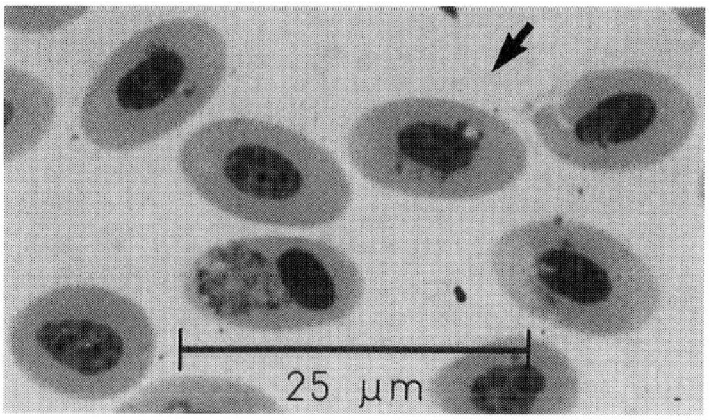

Figure 5.8 Maturing schizont, above left side of scale bar, same parasite and slide as Figure 5.6; in mixed infection with *P. (N.) nucleophilum*, of which a binucleate schizont is arrowed at upper right.

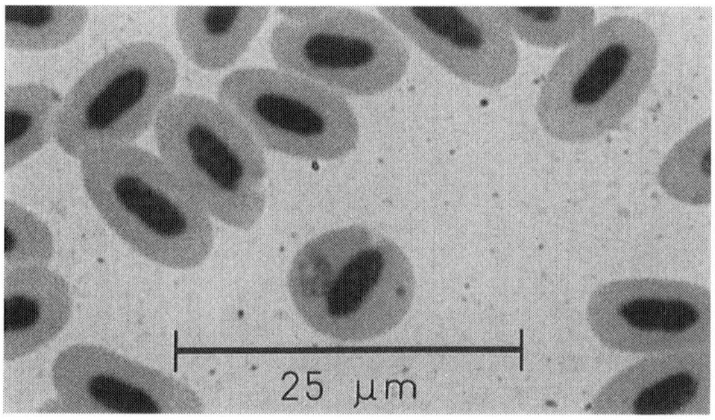

Figure 5.9 *P. (H.) matutinum* ex *Lanius cristatus*, newly invaded merozoite at right of erythroblast, developing trophozoite at left; Aborlan, Palawan, Philippines, 8 April 1963.

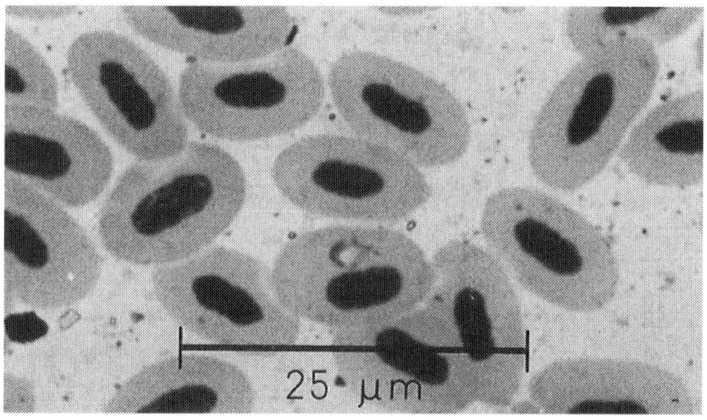

Figure 5.10 *P. (H.) matutinum* ex *Lonchura malacca*, developing trophozoite displacing nucleus of hypertrophied erythrocyte; Subang, Malaysia, 19 December 1962.

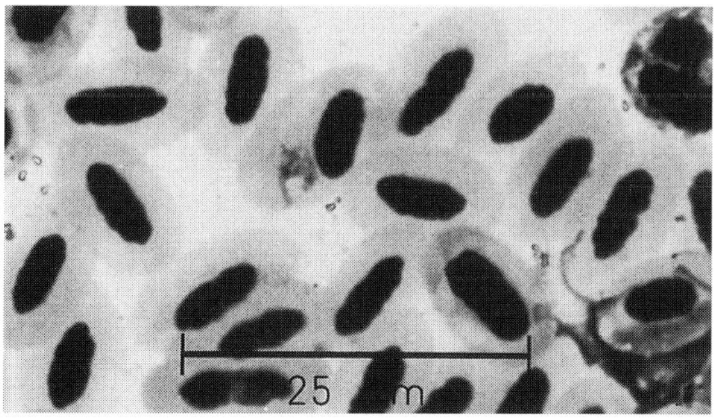

Figure 5.11 *P. (H.) matutinum* ex *Copsychus saularis*, showing further displacement, with tilting, of nucleus of hypertrophied erythrocyte; Rantau Panjang, Malaysia, 6 January 1961.

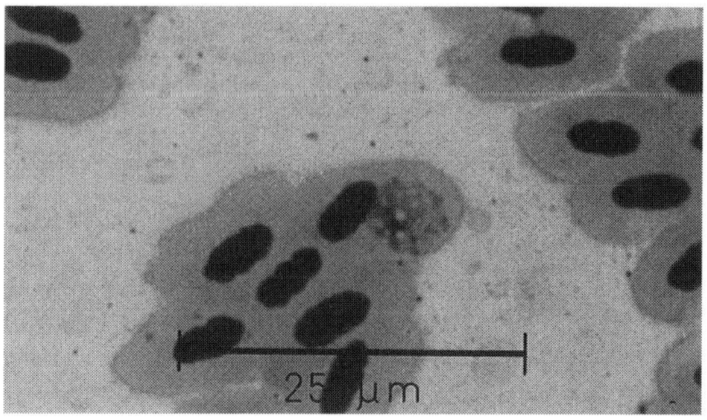

Figure 5.12 *P. (H.) matutinum* ex *Lonchura malacca*, "punched out" vacuoles in developing schizont; Subang, Malaysia, 19 December 1962.

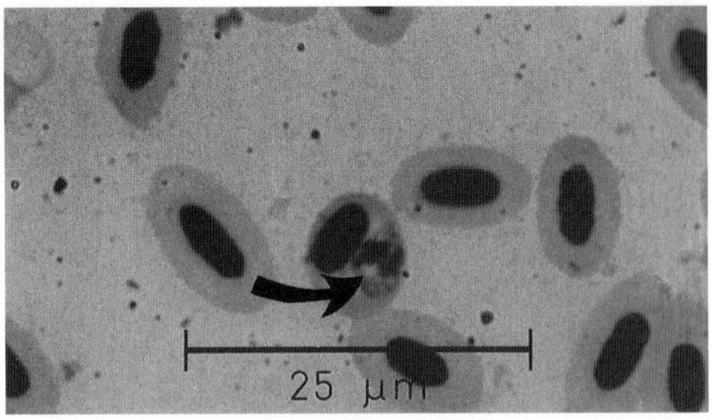

Figure 5.13 *P. (H.) matutinum* ex *Luscinia cyane*, "punched out" vacuole in a schizont, host-cell nucleus displaced to corpuscle's periphery (arrowed); Subang, Malaysia, 7 November 1962.

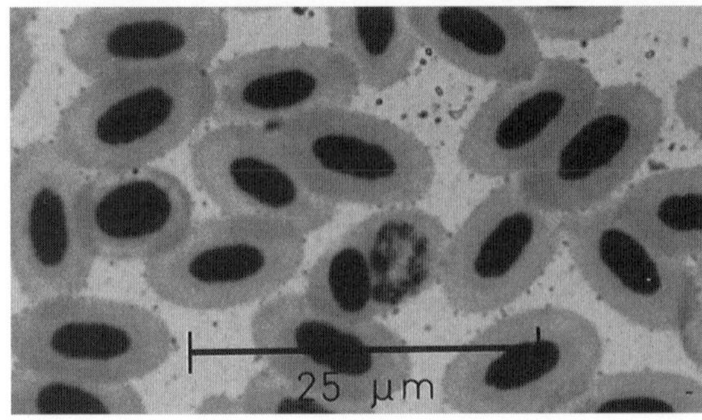

Figure 5.14 *P. (H.) matutinum* ex *Ploceus philippinus*, octonucleate schizont; Bang Phra, Cholburi, Thailand, 1 September 1966.

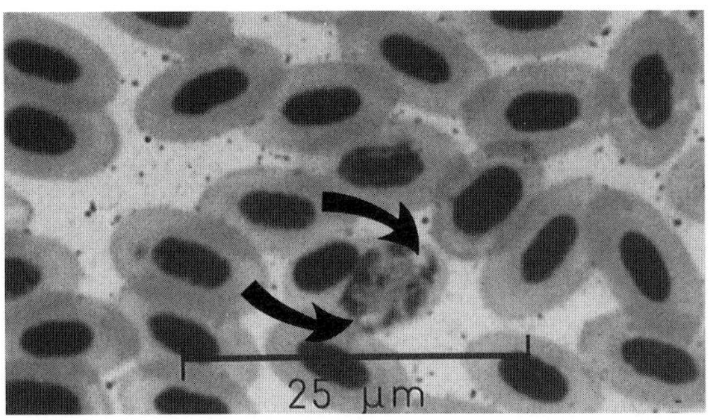

Figure 5.15 Same species and slide as last, maturing schizont with eight mostly peripheral nuclei, and persisting "punched out" vacuoles (arrowed).

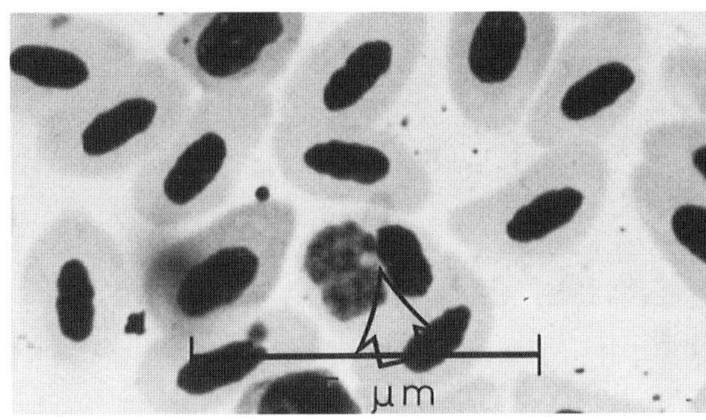

Figure 5.16 *P. (H.) matutinum* ex *Copsychus saularis*, maturing 14-nucleate schizont, and "punched out" vacuole (arrowed); Mahabaleshwar, India, 31 March 1960.

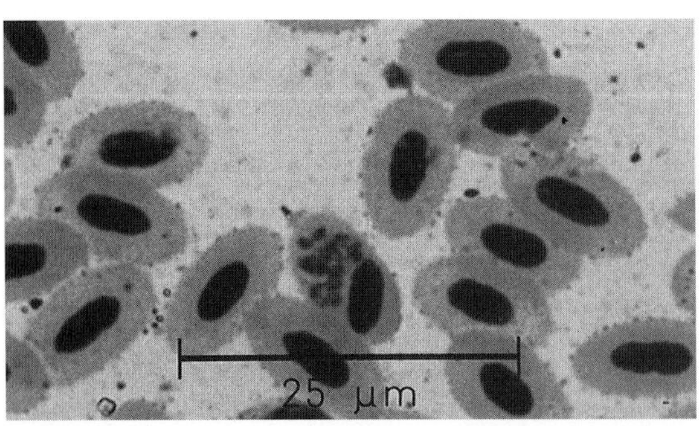

Figure 5.17 *P. (H.) matutinum* ex *Ploceus philippinus*, 12-merozoite segmenter; Bang Phra, Cholburi, Thailand, 1 September 1966.

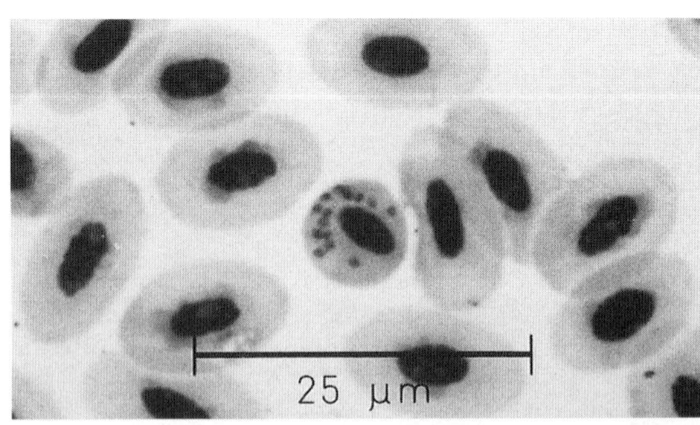

Figure 5.18 *P. (H.) matutinum* ex *Nectarinia jugularis* (with *P. (G.) polare* in joint infection), 14 dispersed merozoites in polychromatophil erythroblast; Tarabanan, Palawan, Philippines, 13 May 1962.

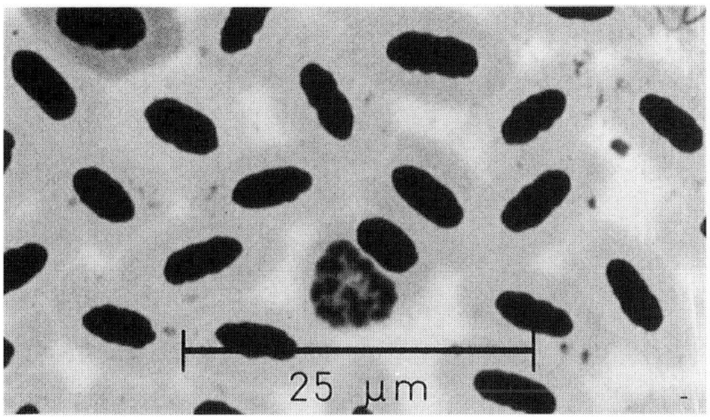

Figure 5.19 *P. (H.) matutinum* ex *Lanius cristatus*, schizont with 16 tightly packed nuclei not yet condensed to final merozoite size, near-central chromatin mass; Subang, Malaysia, 21 July 1962.

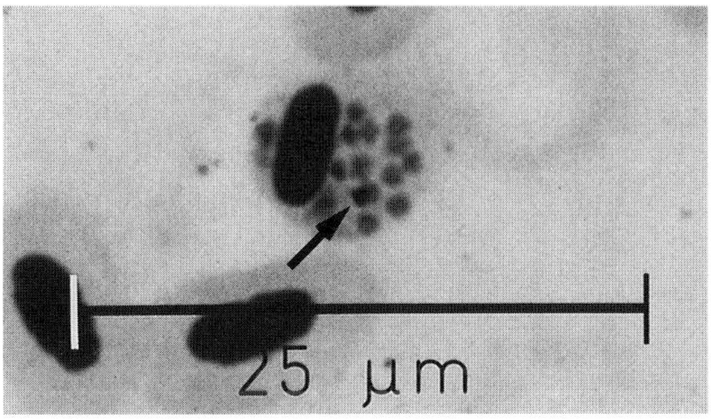

Figure 5.20 Same species and slide as Figure 5.18, merozoites not yet fully condensed, typical pigment concentration arrowed, host-cell nucleus radically displaced.

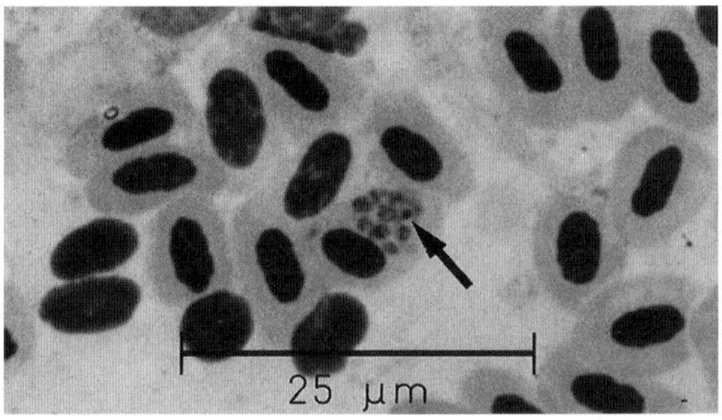

Figure 5.21 Same species and slide as Figure 5.19, eight+ separating merozoites, pigment mass arrowed.

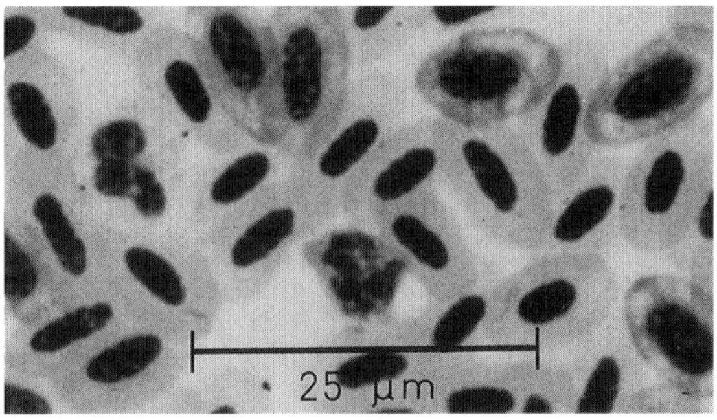

Figure 5.22 *P. (H.) matutinum* ex *Trichastoma rostratum*, maturing schizont with approximately 14 crowded nuclei within enucleated red cell; Rantau Panjang, Malaysia, 8 March 1960.

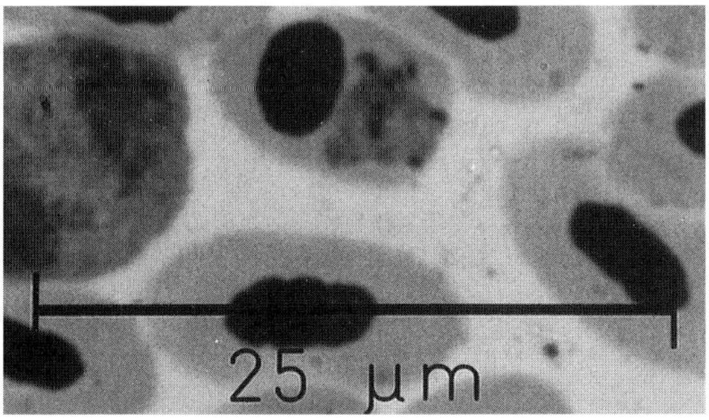

Figure 5.23 *P. (H.) matutinum* ex *Lonchura malacca*, early gametocyte with scalloped outline and pigment granules mostly peripheral; Subang, Malaysia, 19 December 1962.

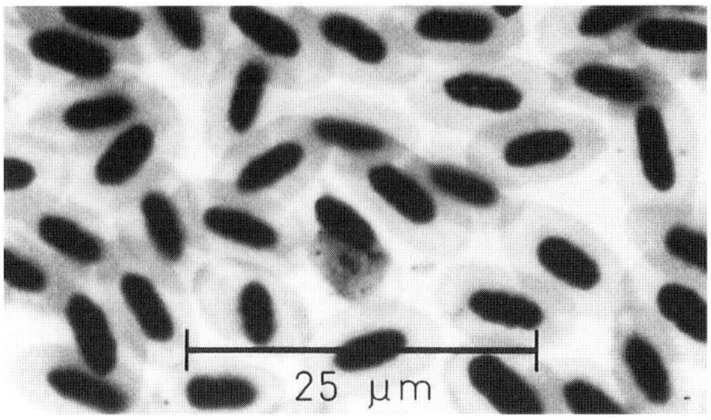

Figure 5.24 *P. (H.) matutinum* ex *Ploceus manyar*, macrogametocyte within erythrocyte with nucleus displaced to periphery; Bangkok, Thailand, 12 March 1967.

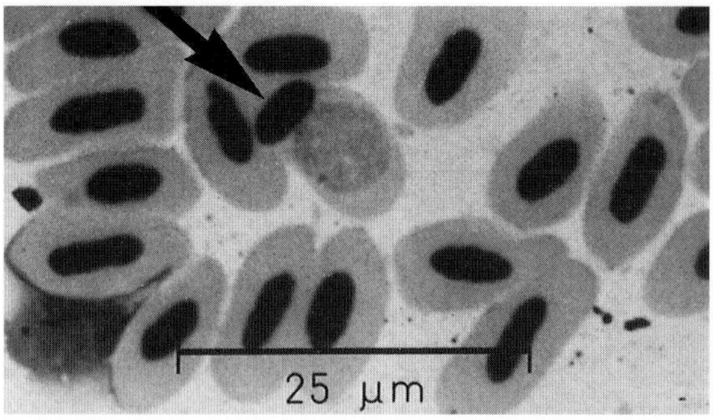

Figure 5.25 *P. (H.) matutinum* ex *Lanius cristatus*, poorly stained and faded microgametocyte within red cell, the (arrowed) nucleus of which is being expelled; Ping-Tung, Taiwan, 15 Sepember 1965.

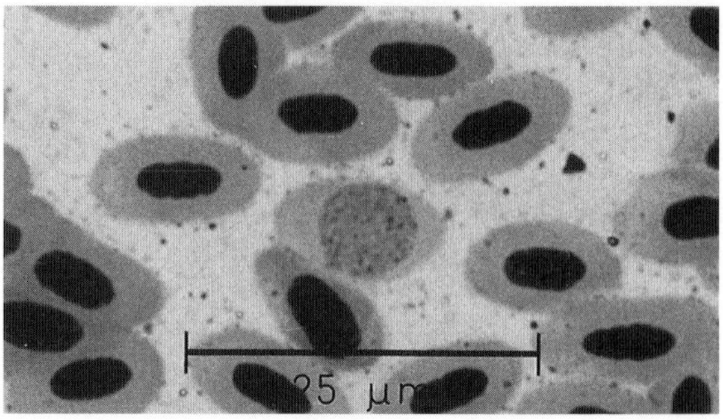

Figure 5.26 *P. (H.) matutinum* ex *Ploceus philippinus*, mature round microgametocyte, within enucleated erythrocyte; Bang Phra, Cholburi, Thailand, 1 September 1966.

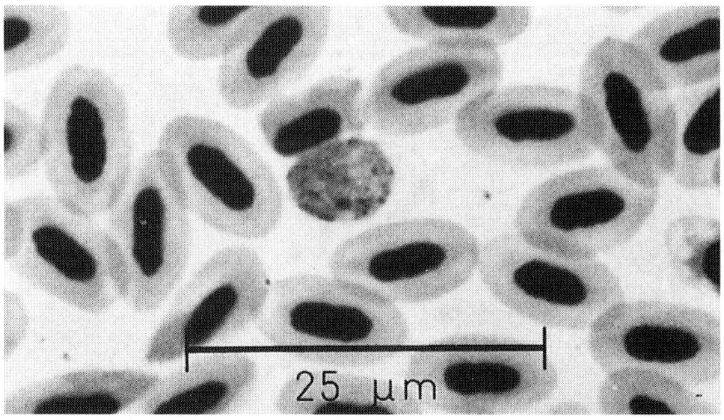

Figure 5.27 *P. (H.) matutinum* ex *Ploceus manyar*, macrogametocyte just freed from the host cell, the membrane of which is retracting about its nucleus, above; Bangkok, Thailand, 12 March 1967.

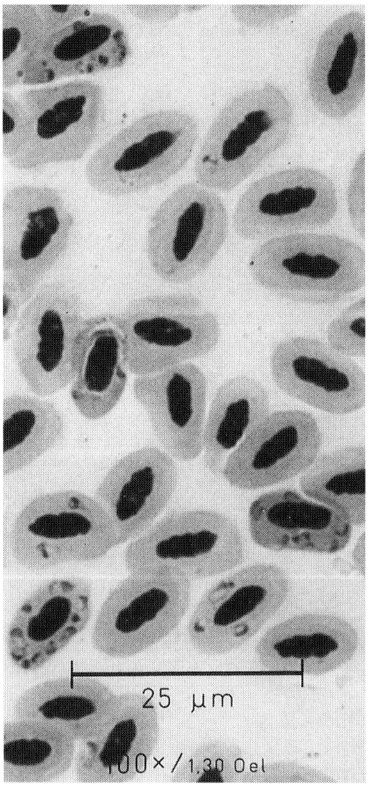

Figure 5.28 *P. (H.) giovannolai (?)* ex *Acrocephalus stentoreus*, individual red cells harbouring up to ten early trophozoites and invasive merozoites; Mahárlú, Iran, 25 June 1967.

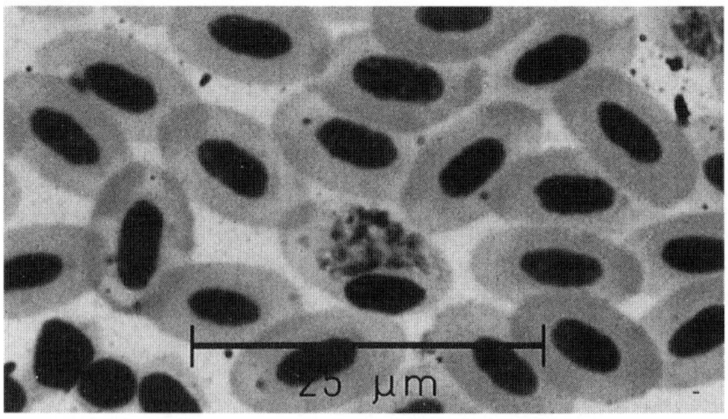

Figure 5.29 *P. (H.) giovannolai (?)* ex *Acrocephalus aedon*, developing schizont; Sara Buri, Thailand, 13 January 1965.

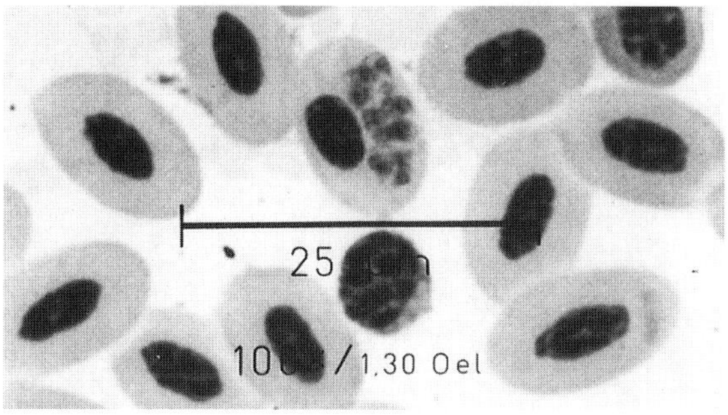

Figure 6.1 *P. (Giovannolaia) fallax* ex *Otus lempiji*, developing schizont (12 nuclei could be differentiated under the microscope); Nakhon Ratchasima, Thailand, 18 September 1967.

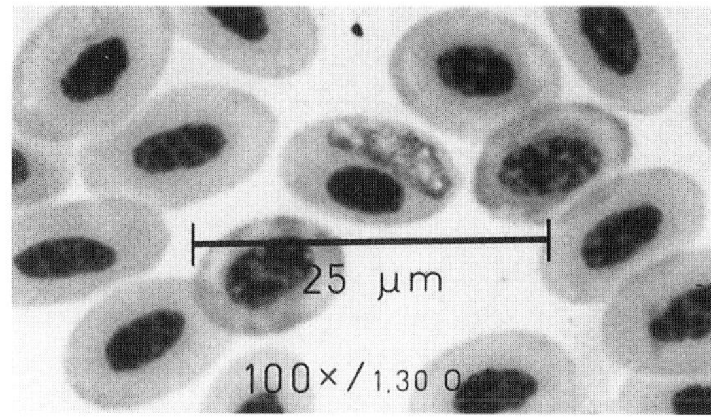

Figure 6.2 Same species and slide as Figure 6.1, characteristically vacuolated early gametocyte laterally displacing host-cell nucleus.

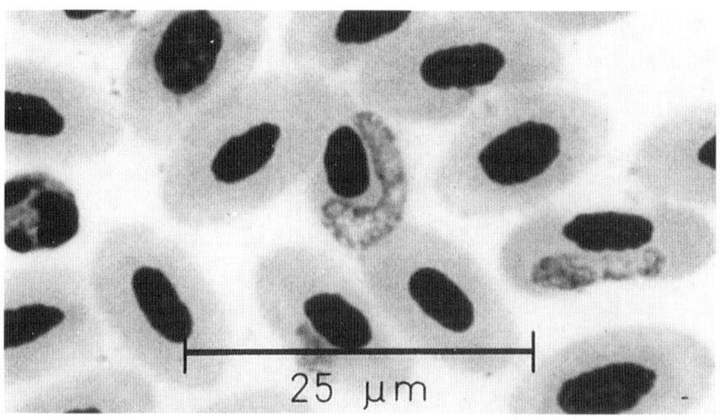

Figure 6.3 *P. (G.) fallax* ex *Otus lempiji*, typical microgametocyte of this parasite with one extremity hooked around the host-cell nucleus; Chiang Mai, Thailand, 2 October 1967.

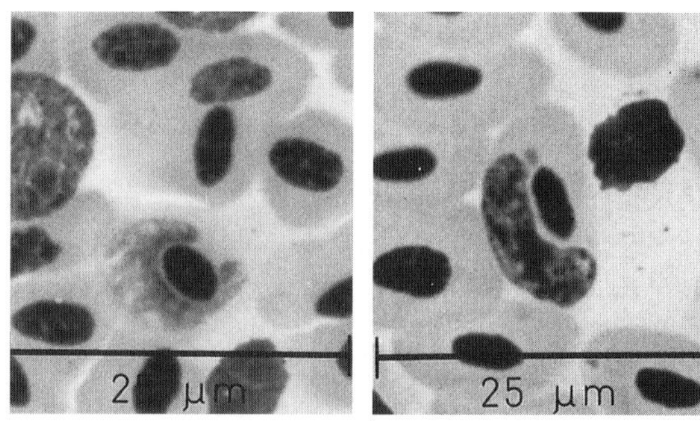

a b

Figure 6.4a *P. (G.) fallax* ex *Ninox philippensis*, microgametocyte; Basay, Negros Oriental, Philippines, 20 December 1964.

Figure 6.4b. *P. (G.) fallax* ex *Ninox philippensis*, macrogametocyte of characteristically hooked form.

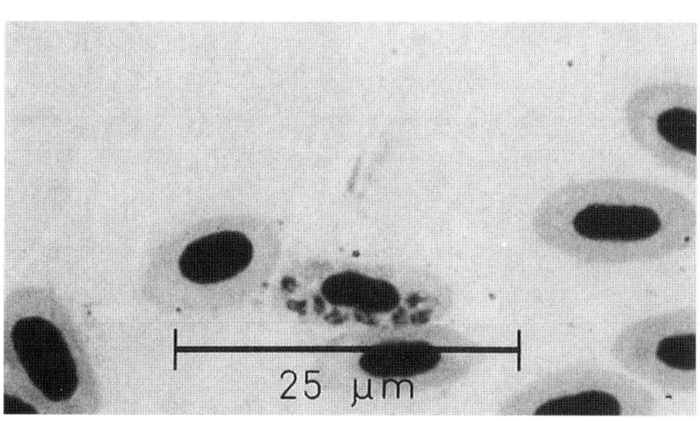

Figure 6.5 *P. (G.) circumflexum* ex *Pycnonotus goiavier*, developing octonucleate schizont; Bang Phra, Thailand, October (date and year unknown due to label damage).

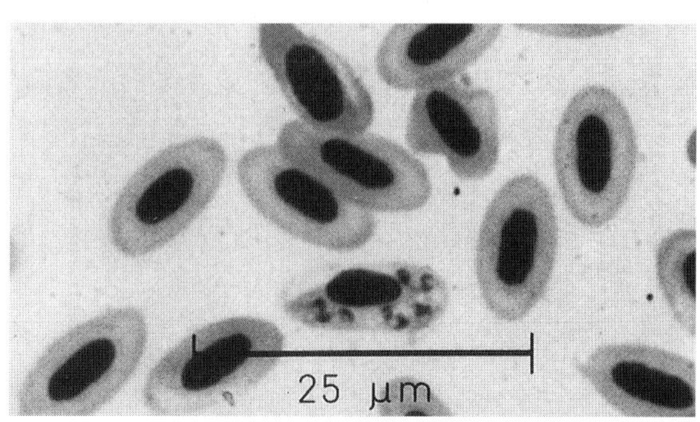

Figure 6.6 *P. (G.) circumflexum* ex *Pycnonotus melanoleucos*, maturing presegmenter with eight developing merozoites; Ban Skaerat, Thailand, 25 June 1967.

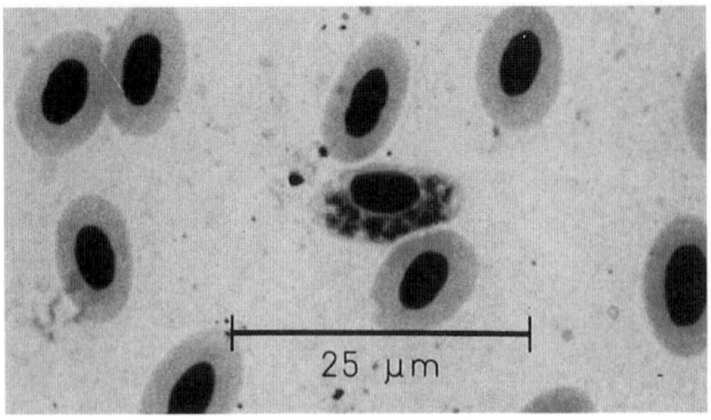

Figure 6.7 *P. (G.) circumflexum* ex *Sturnus nigricollis*, up to 16 tightly packed, condensed merozoites; Bang Phra, Thailand, 27 December 1967.

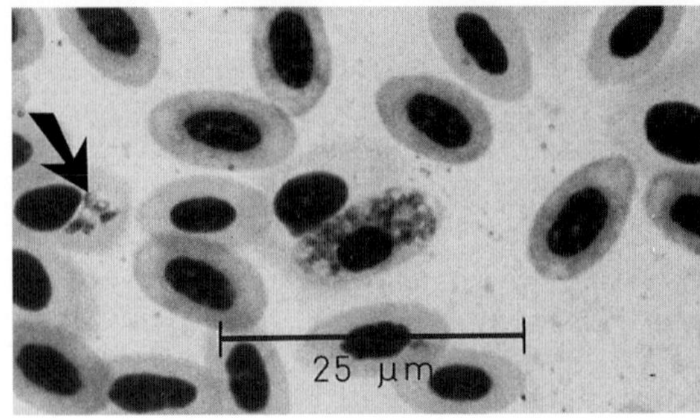

Figure 6.8 Same species and slide as Figure 6.7, staining of central segmenter faded, but 18 merozoites were distinguishable by microscopy using maximum light; arrow at left indicates a hexanucleate schizont of *P. (Novyella) nucleophilum* pulled away from host-cell nucleus during smearing.

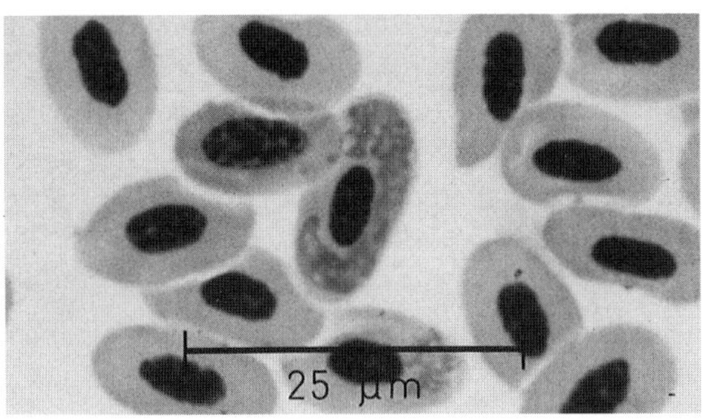

Figure 6.9 *Haemoproteus pastoris*, same slide as Figures 6.7 and 6.8, faded gametocyte.

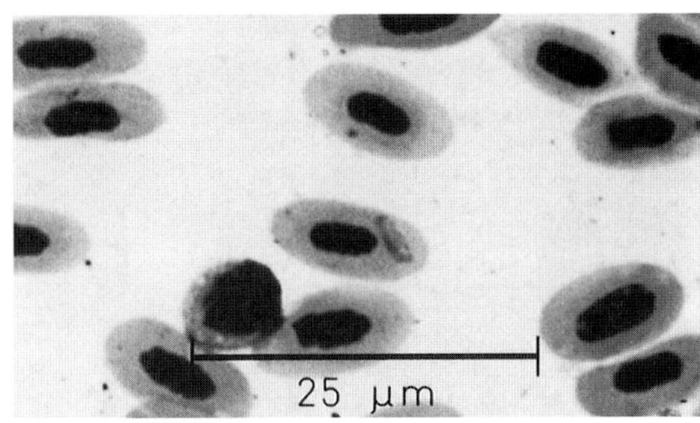

Figure 6.10 *P. (G.) polare* ex *Pycnonotus melanicterus*, young polar trophozoite; Mt Brinchang, Malaysia, 18 March 1960.

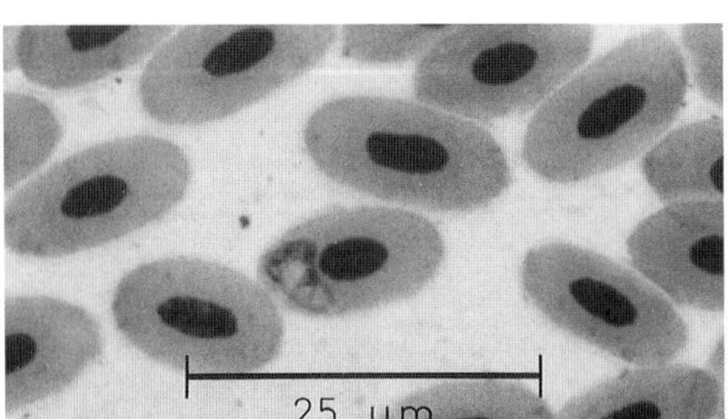

Figure 6.11 *P. (G.) polare* ex *Amaurornis phoenicurus* (pure infection), developing polar schizont; Subang, Malaysia, 29 November 1962.

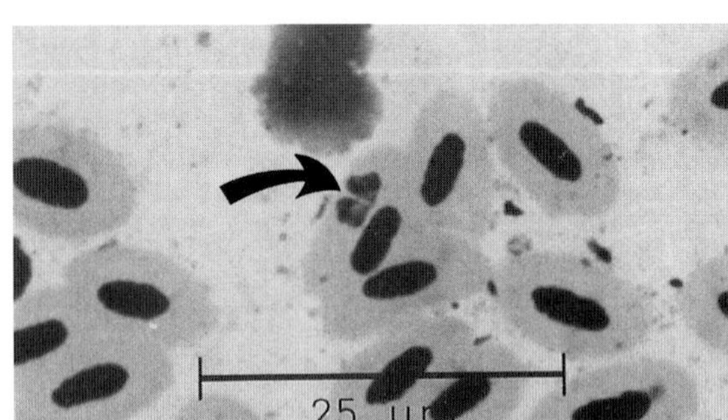

Figure 6.12 *P. (G.) polare* ex *Dicrurus annectans*, penultimate division of schizont nuclei; *P. (N.) vaughani* was in joint infection. The latter's hexanucleate segmenters (Figure 7.5, left-hand example) being decidedly smaller than those of this figure; Subang, Malaysia, 25 October 1962.

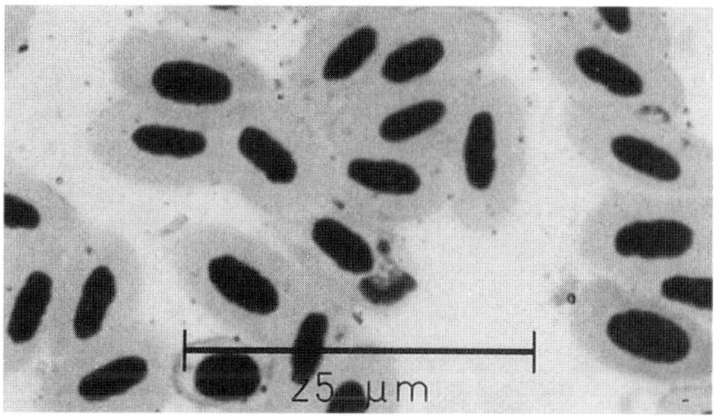

Figure 6.13 *P. (G.) polare* ex *Anthreptes malacensis*, schizont fan of eight large and intensely stained nuclei, separated from the discrete pigment mass at distal end of "handle" by prominent and conspicuously vacuolated cytoplasm; Rantau Panjang, Malaysia, 2 May 1965.

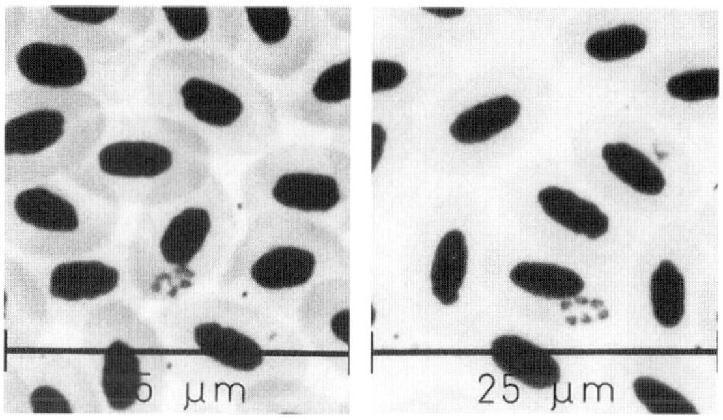

a b

Figure 6.14a *P. (N.) vaughani* ex *Zoothera sibirica* (joint infection with *P. rouxi*), polar schizont with six nuclei; Mt Brinchang, Malaysia, January 1965.

Figure 6.14b *P. (N.) vaughani* ex *Stachyris poliocephala*, segmenter with six condensing merozoites (compare Figure 7.5); Kuala Lumpur, Malaysia, 9 January 1965.

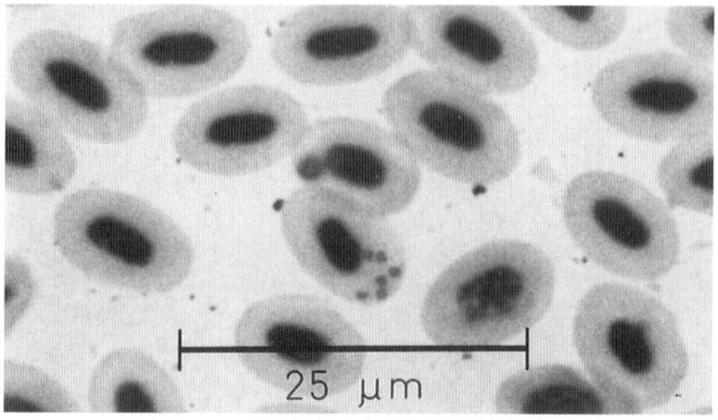

Figure 6.15 *P. (N.) vaughani* ex *Pycnonotus melanoleucus*, six condensed and dispersed merozoites; Nakhon Ratchasima, Thailand, 28 June 1967.

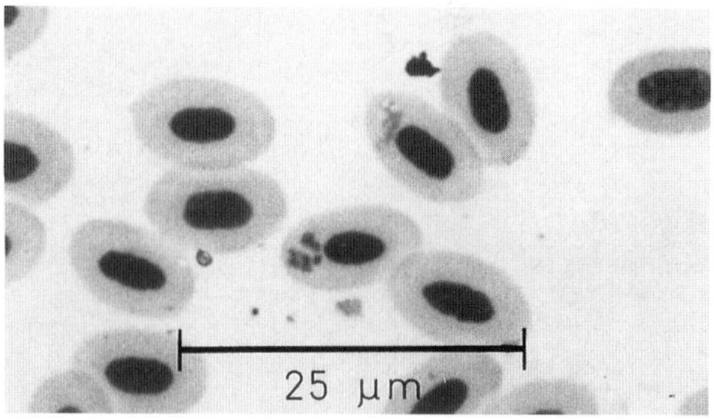

Figure 6.16 Same species and slide as Figure 6.15, putative octonucleate schizont with its uppermost chromatin mass still to divide.

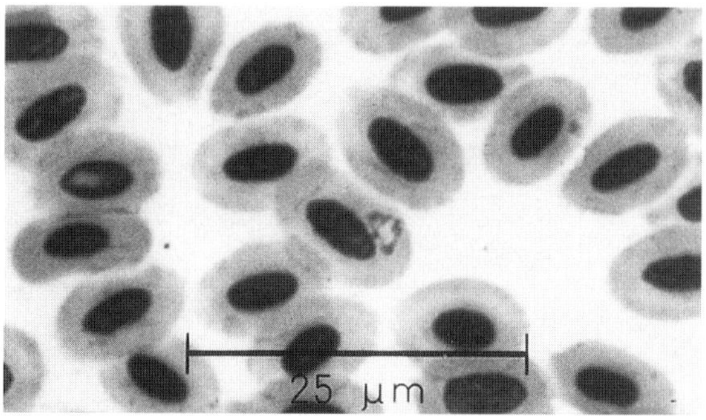

Figure 6.17 *P. (N.) vaughani* ex *Pycnonotus plumosus*, quadrinucleate schizont fan with relatively plentiful cytoplasm (much less of which is evident in *P. (N.) rouxi*, which was in joint infection); Iwahig, Palawan, Philippines, 30 March 1965.

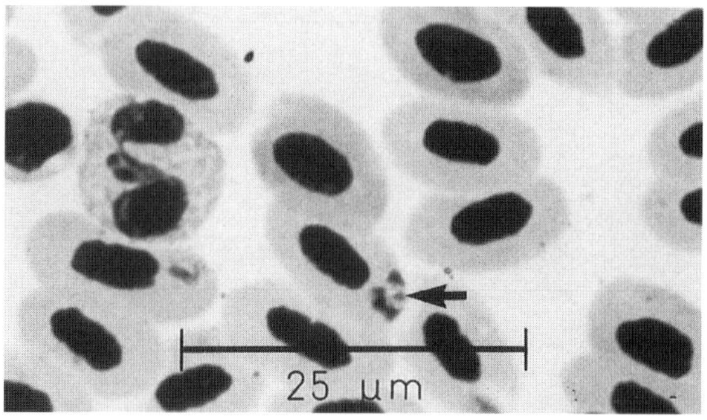

Figure 6.18 *P. (N.) vaughani* in *Copsychus saularis* (pure infection), quadrinucleate presegmenter, the developing merozoites of the typically triangular shape ensured by the fan configuration; Rantau Panjang, Malaysia, 11 August 1962.

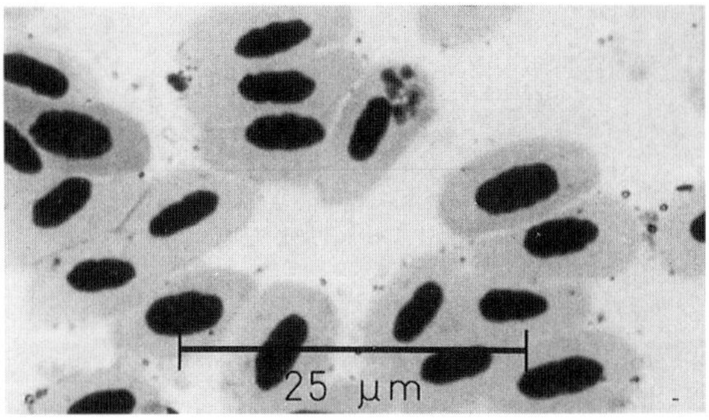

Figure 6.19 *P. (G.) polare* ex *Trichastoma rostratum* (pure infection), polar schizont with six chromatin masses each destined for a further division, and three bright little vacuoles in central cytoplasm; Rantau Panjang, Malaysia, 8 October 1960.

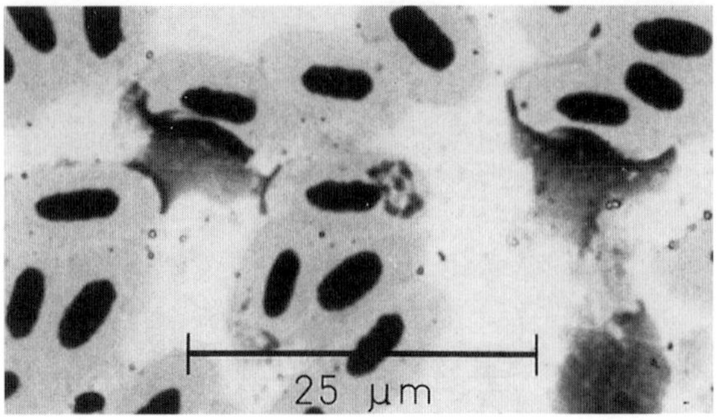

Figure 6.20 *P. (G.) polare* ex, same slide as Figure 6.13, polar schizont with eight developing merozoites, and characteristically "stranded" cytoplasm.

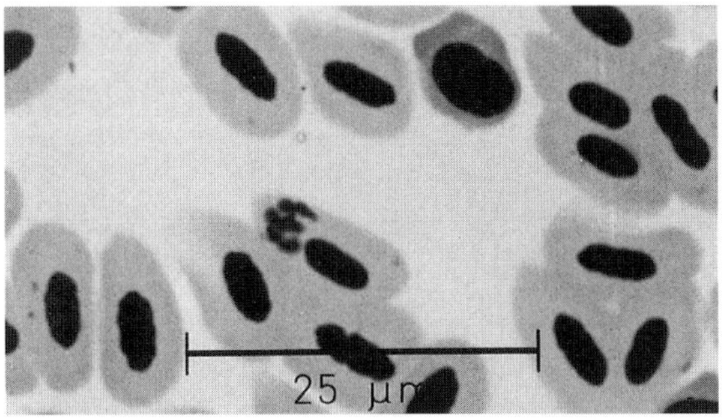

Figure 6.21 *P. (G.) polare* ex, same slide as Figure 6.12, octonucleate segmenter with cytoplasm no longer evident, but with the pyriform products of a schizont fan still to round up as merozoites.

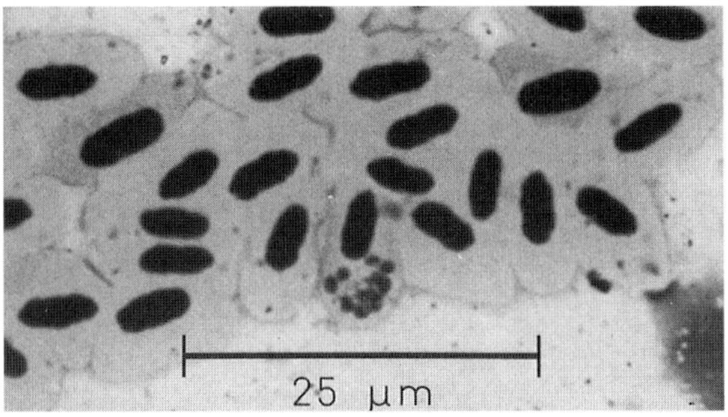

Figure 6.22 *P. (G.) polare* ex *Amaurornis phoenicurus*, segmenter with ten condensing merozoites; Rantau Panjang, Malaysia, 20 May 1960.

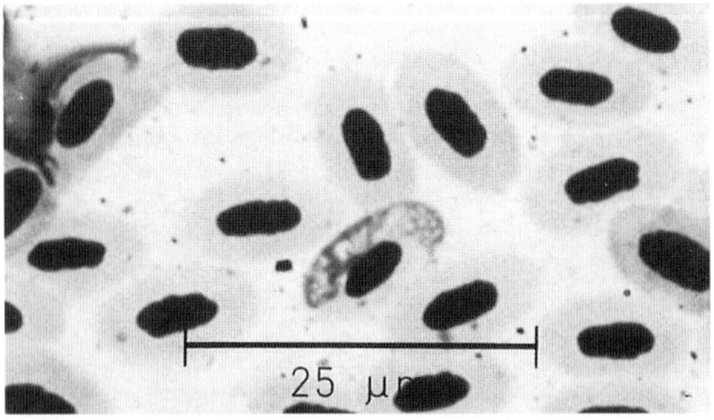

Figure 6.23 *P. (G.) polare* ex *Ploceus philippinus*, macrogametocyte with terminal finger-like projection; Sungei Way, Selangor, Malaysia, 24 January 1963.

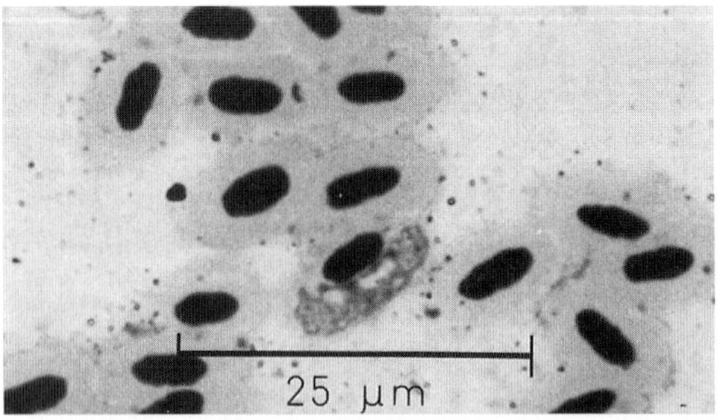

Figure 6.24 *P. (G.) polare*, same slide as Figure 6.26, mature gametocyte with conspicuously irregular outline.

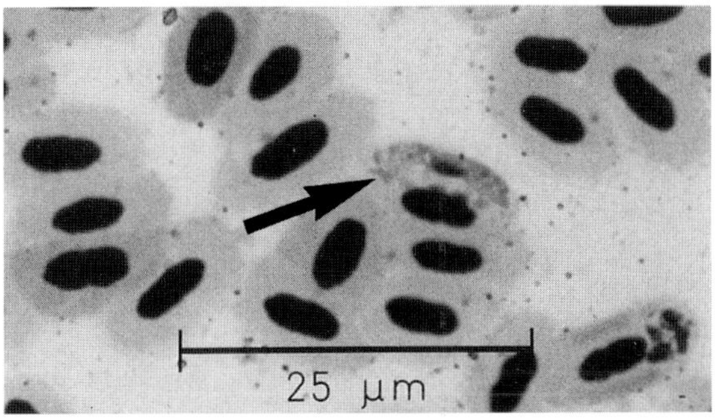

Figure 6.25 *P. (G.) polare*, same slide as Figures 6.24 and 6.26, marginal fimbriations of mature gametocyte arrowed. Note how these protrusions project into the host-cell nucleus.

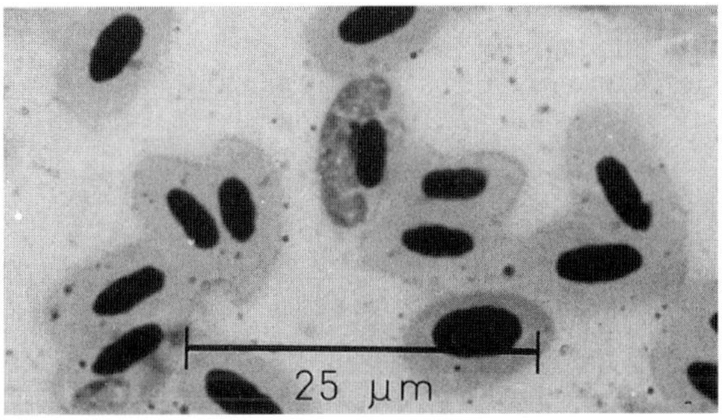

Figure 6.26 *Haemoproteus sequeirae* ex joint infection with *P. polare*, same slide as Figure 6.13; its entire margin and particularly the smoothly rounded ends of the gametocyte, distinguishing it from the latter species' often irregularly margined sexual stages as seen in Figures 6.23–6.25.

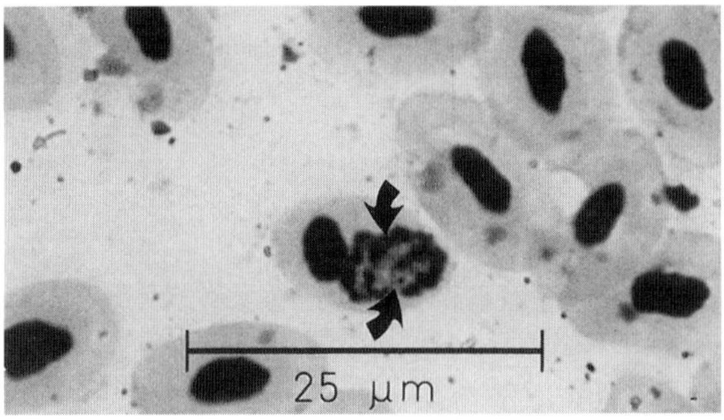

Figure 6.27 Same slide as Figure 6.29, *Plasmodium* **incertae sedis** double occupancy of a corpuscle (its nucleus displaced and tilted) by two octonucleate schizonts, their line of demarcation arrowed. Joint infection with *P. lophurae.*

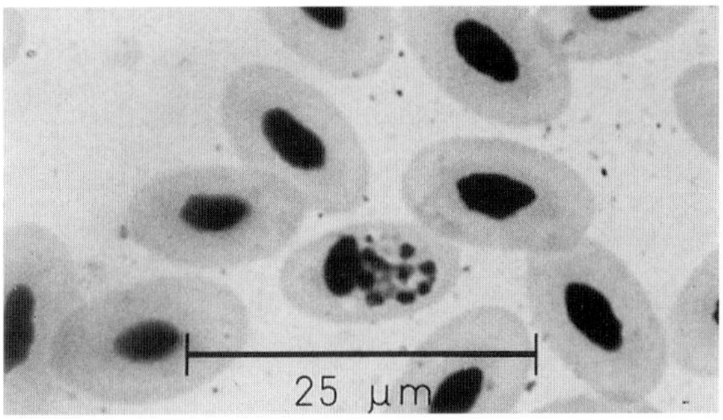

Figure 6.28 Same slide as Figure 6.27, *Plasmodium* **incertae sedis** octonucleate segmenter; nucleus of host red cell displaced and tilted.

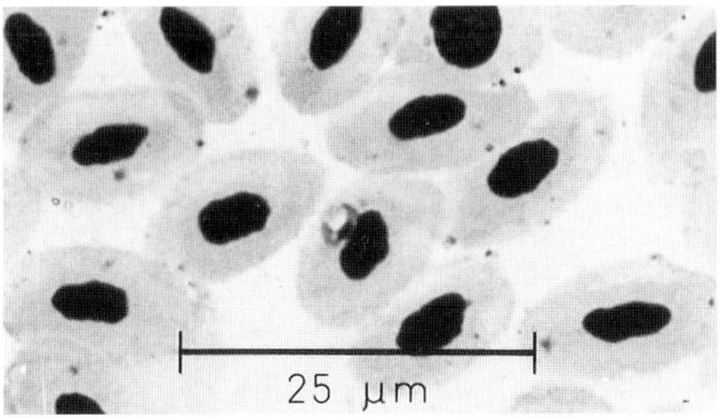

Figure 6.29 *P. (G.) lophurae* ex *Lophura erythropthalma*, developing trophozoite with conspicuous vacuole; Subang, Malaysia, 25 October 1963

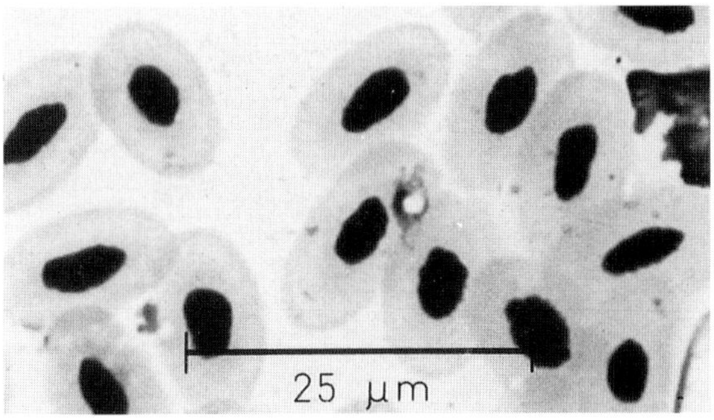

Figure 6.30 Same species and slide as Figure 6.29, brightly vacuolate late trophozoite.

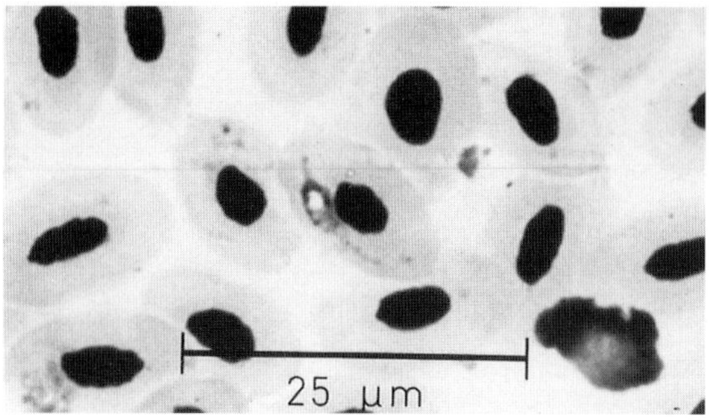

Figure 6.31 Same species and slide as Figures 6.29 and 6.30, developing schizont with terminal filopodia, the lowermost at 4.7 μm accounting for 46% of the organism's overall length; Siaton, Negros Oriental, Philippines, 17 February 1965.

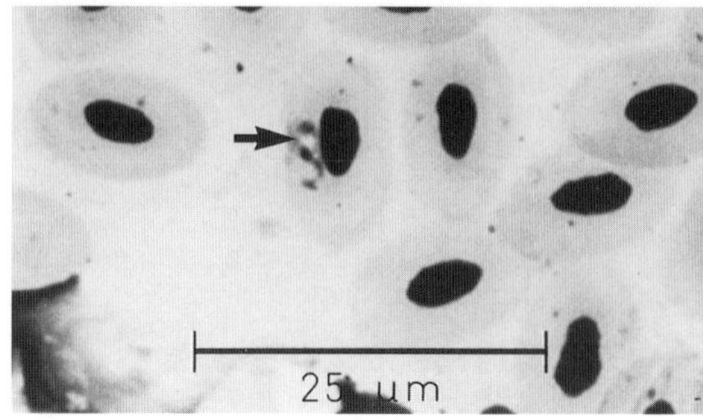

Figure 6.32 Same slide as Figures 6.29–6.31, *P. (G.) lophurae*, early division of schizont chromatin with one of two "orange vacuoles" arrowed.

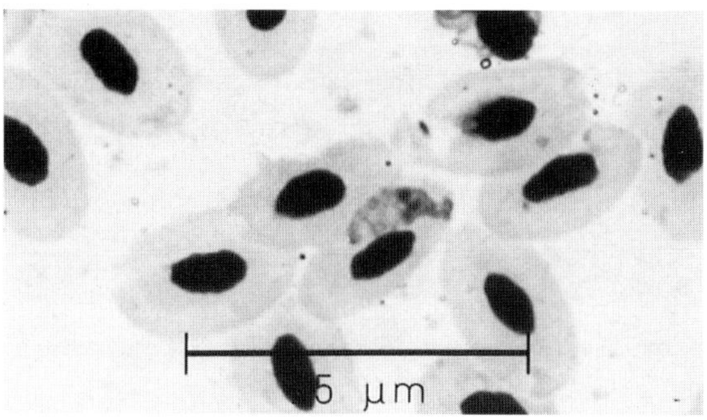

Figure 6.33 Same species and slide as Figure 6.29, developing schizont.

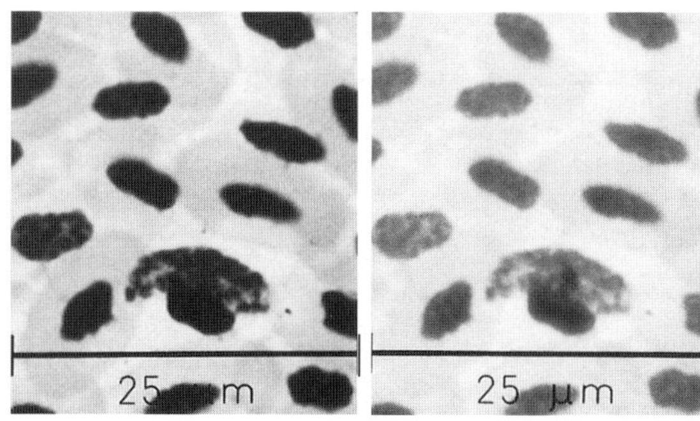

a b

Figure 6.34a Same species and slide as Figure 6.29, segmenter with 18 condensing merozoites too deeply stained and crowded for counting as photographed, but distinguishable by direct phase-contrast microscopy.

Figure 6.34b Same segmenter as Figure 6.34a, this time photographed using a blue filter to emphasize the central patch of dark brown pigment.

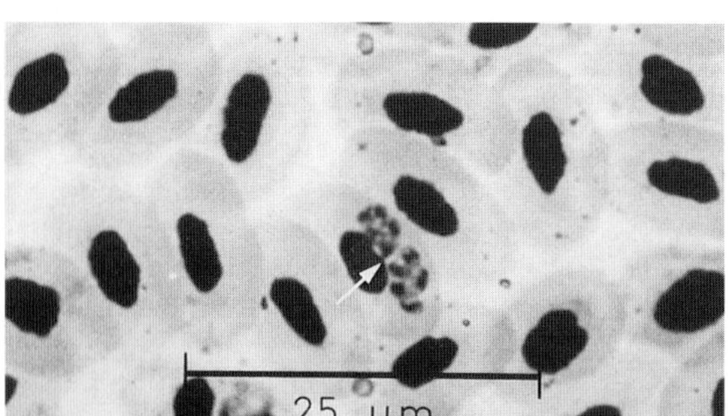

Figure 6.35 Same species and slide as Figure 6.29, a ten-merozoite segmenter with pigment patch arrowed.

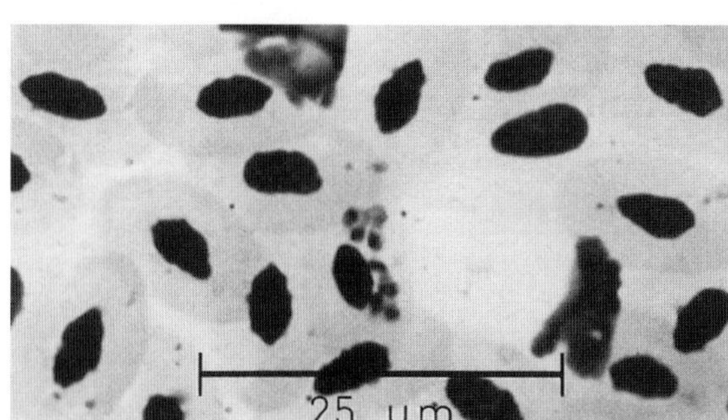

Figure 6.36 Same species and slide as Figure 6.29, not a double occupancy of a mature erythrocyte by quadrinucleate schizonts, but an octonucleate segmenter parting into two sections.

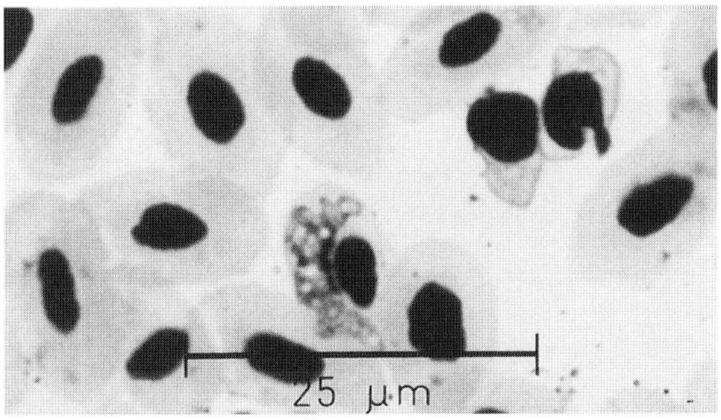

Figure 6.37 Same species and slide as Figure 6.29, mature macrogametocyte exhibiting vacuolation and prominently rugose outer margin.

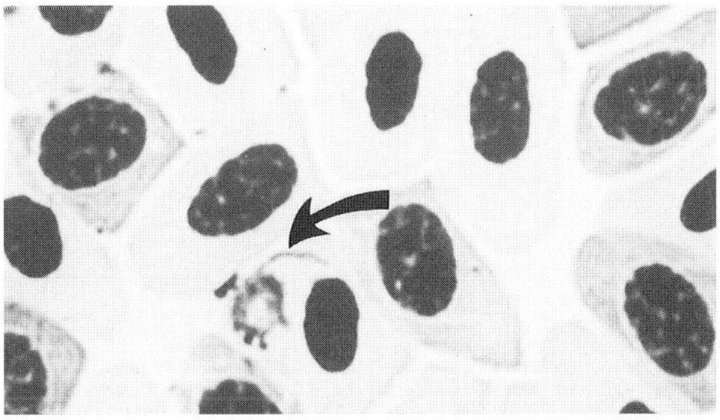

Figure 6.38 *P. (G.) dissanaikei* ex *Amaurornis phoenicurus*, amoeboid trophozoite with distinctively long filopodium arrowed (a 25 μm scale-bar for this illustration and Figures 6.39 and 6.42–6.45 would measure 59 mm, as does that for Figure 7.28); Subang, Malaysia, 28 August 1962.

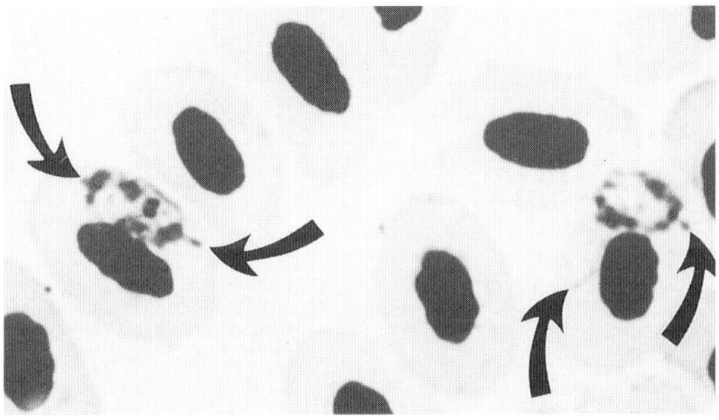

Figure 6.39 Same parasite and slide as Figure 6.38, early schizont at right, filopodia arrowed; as are those of the common later stage seen at left.

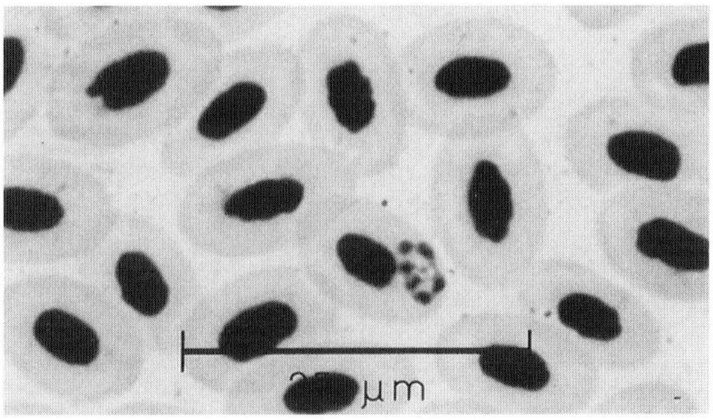

Figure 6.40 *P. (N.) nucleophilum*, same doubly parasitized slide as Figure 6.38, hexanucleate schizont and central dot of yellowish-brown pigment.

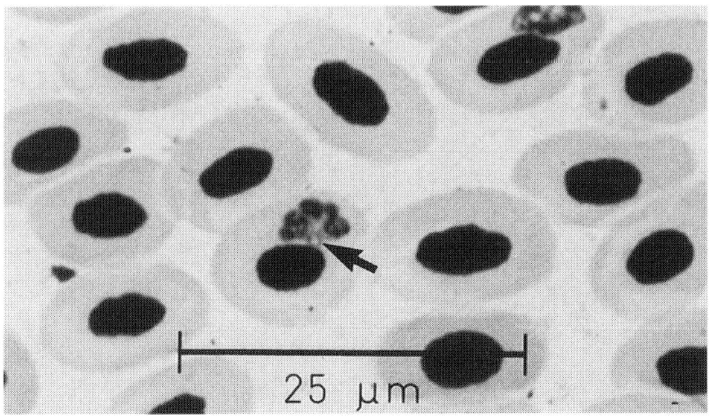

Figure 6.41 *P. (G.) dissanaikei*, same slide as Figure 6.38, schizont with six massive and deeply stained nuclei, little cytoplasm evident and a circular refractile globule at the fan's "handle".

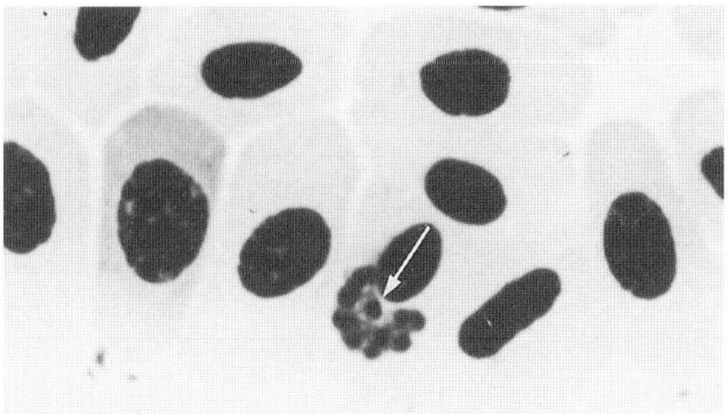

Figure 6.42 Same species and slide as Figure 6.38, ten-merozoite polar segmenter in horseshoe formation, the central mass of yellowish-brown pigment arrowed.

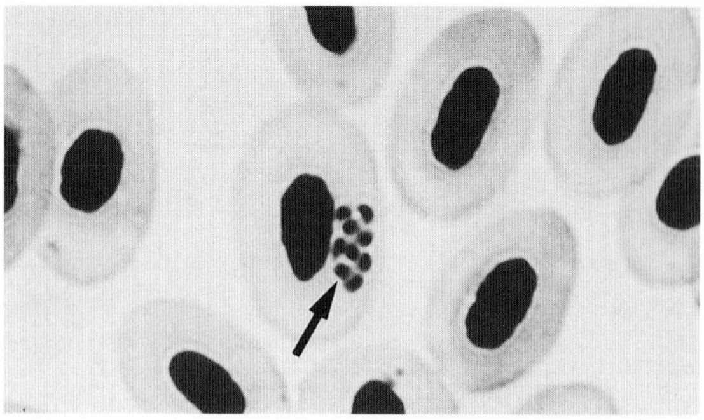

Figure 6.43 Same species and slide as Figure 6.38, laterally oriented segmenter with eight condensing merozoites, pigment mass arrowed.

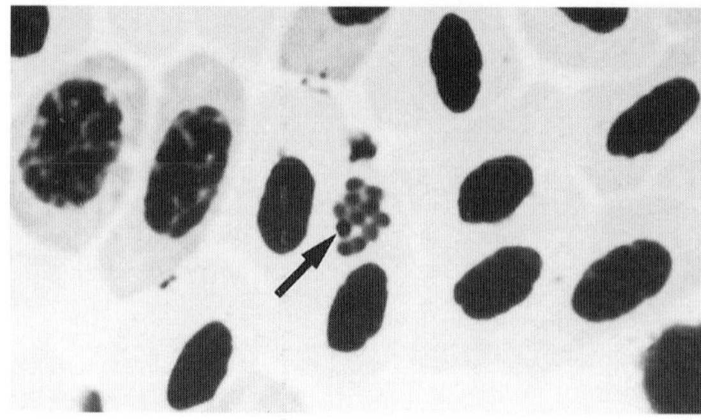

Figure 6.44 Same species and slide as Figure 6.38, latero-polar segmenter with ten fully condensed merozoites, pigment mass arrowed, and host-cell nucleus displaced towards opposite pole.

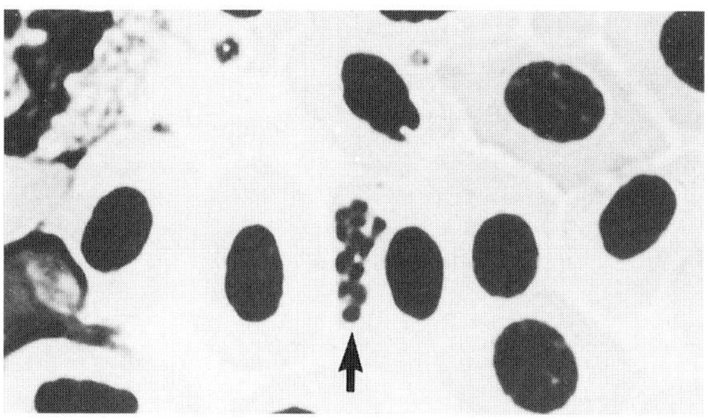

Figure 6.45 Same species and slide as Figure 6.38, segmenter with 12 fully condensed merozoites alongside laterally displaced host-cell nucleus, terminal pigment arrowed.

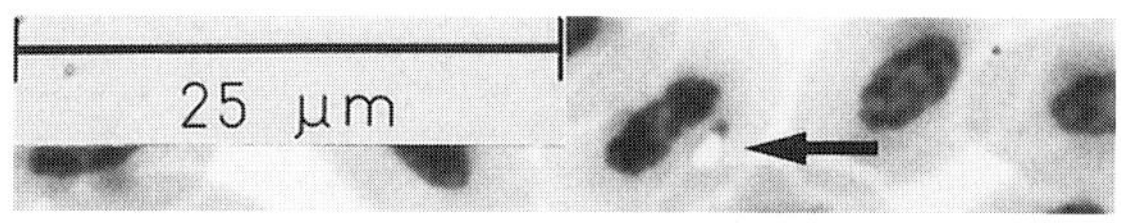

a

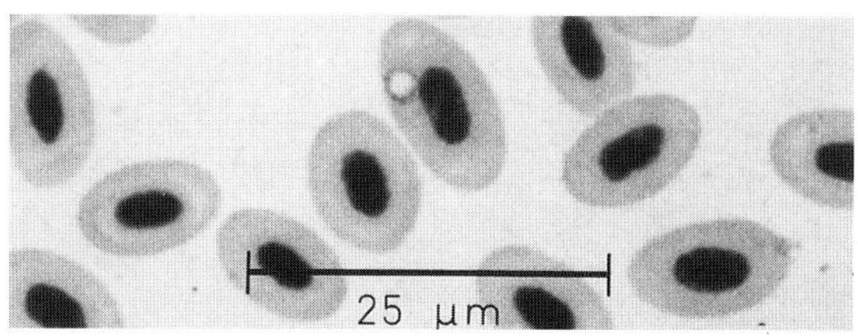

b

Figure 7.1a *P. (N.) vaughani* ex *Rallina euryzonoides* also parasitized by *P. (N.) nucleophilum*, (for the distinctive little rings of which see Figures 7.2 and 7.3), oval trophozoite arrowed; Dalton Pass, Luzon, Philippines, 10 July 1966.

Figure 7.1b *P. (N.) vaughani* ex *Pycnonotus blanfordi*, typical signet-ring trophozoite; Koh Kred, Thailand, 4 August 1964.

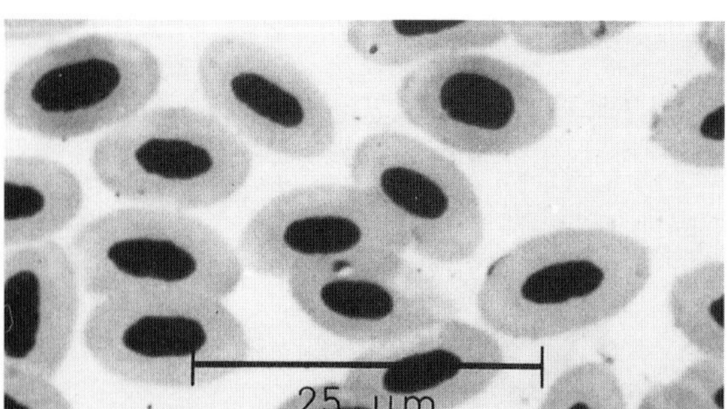

Figure 7.2 Same species and slide as Figure 7.21, signet-ring trophozoite about to contact host-cell nucleus.

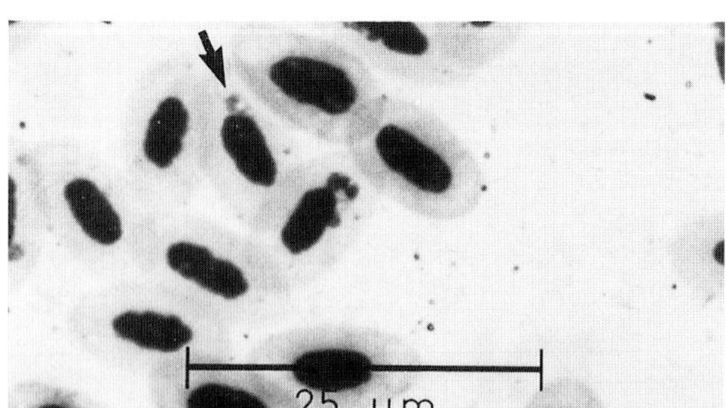

Figure 7.3 *P. (N.) nucleophilum* ex *Sturnus nigricollis* (multiple infection with *P. (G.) circumflexum* and *Haemoproteus pastoris*), signet-ring trophozoite touching a tangential "shoulder" of host-cell nucleus, arrowed; at centre a nucleophilic schizont with four prominent chromatin masses and evident cytoplasm; Bang Phra, Cholburi, Thailand 27 December 1967.

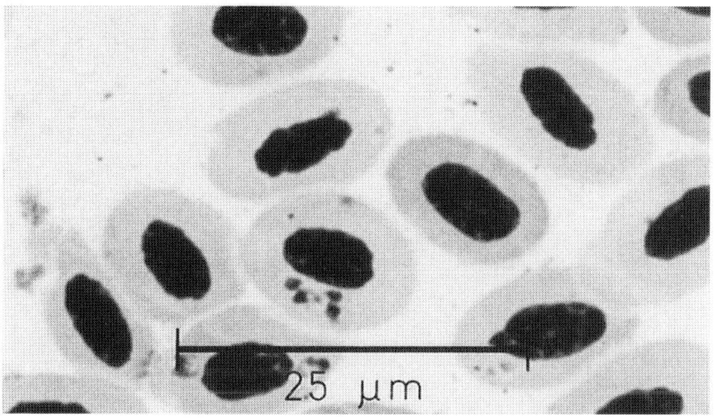

Figure 7.4 *P. (N.) vaughani* ex *Copsychus saularis*, such cruciform presegmenters of *P. vaughani* are often confused with those of *P. rouxi*; these, however, have even scantier cytoplasm, less pigment, and tinier merozoites *never* exceeding four in number (see Figures 7.6a, 7.7b, 7.15).

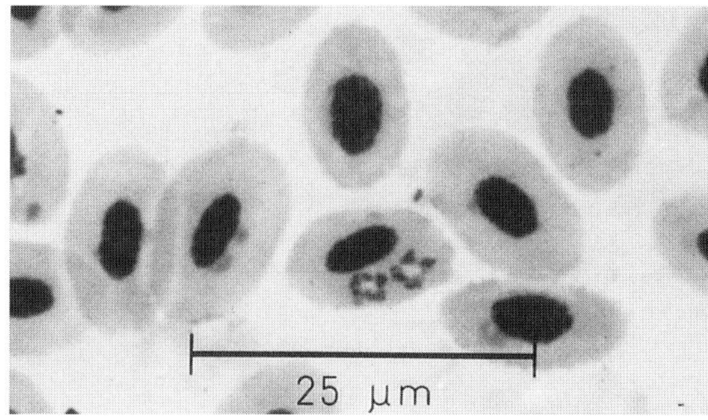

Figure 7.5 Same parasite and slide as Figure 7.4, showing two segmenters (of four and six merozoites) with ample cytoplasm.

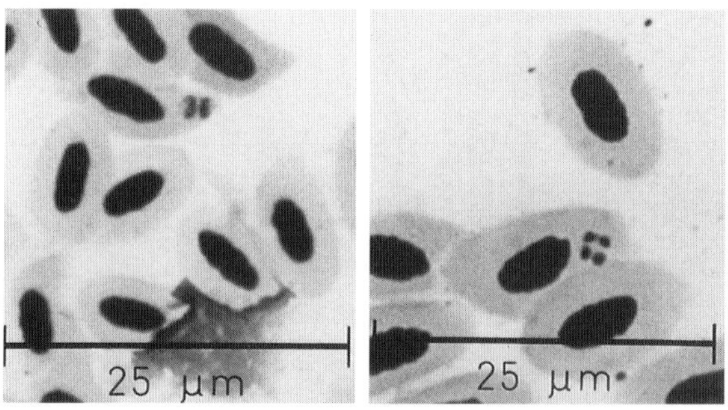

a b

Figure 7.6a *P. (N.) rouxi* ex same slides as Figures 7.12 and 7.13, quadrangular segmenter, the four merozoites condensing and no trace of cytoplasm or pigment (compare *P. vaughani*, Figure 7.8a).

Figure 7.6b *P. corradettii* n.sp. (same slides as Figures 3.1 and 7.7a), quadrangular segmenter with fully condensed and unseparated merozoites, neither cytoplasm nor pigment granules showing. However, the central space was suffused with fading pigment that would have been evident in a colour illustration (see Figure 7.6a).

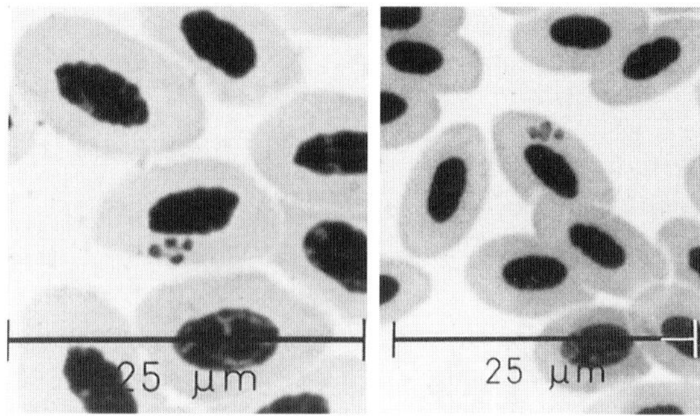

a b

Figure 7.7a *P. (N.) corradettii* n.sp., same slide as Figure 3.1, cruciform schizont with central zone entirely pale brownish-gold (compare *P. vaughani*, Figure 7.4 nuclei larger but still have to condense into spherical merozoites).

Figure 7.7b *P. (N) rouxi* ex *Hypsipetes leucocephalus*, segmenter (at slightly lower magnification than last) lacking both cytoplasm and pigment; Chiang Mai, Thailand, 31 October 1964.

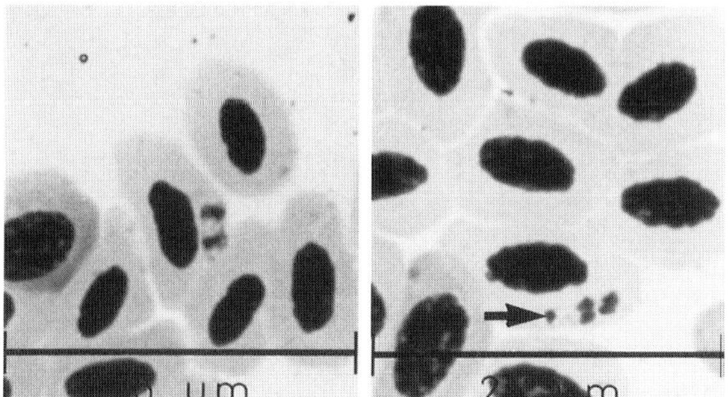

a b

Figure 7.8a *P. (N.) vaughani*, same slide as Figures 6.18, 7.4, 7.5, common quadrangular or box-form of quadrinucleate schizont.

Figure 7.8b *P. (N.) corradettii* n.sp. ex *Pitta moluccensis*, same slide as Figure 3.1, quadrinucleate schizont with terminal (discoidal) pigment plaque arrowed.

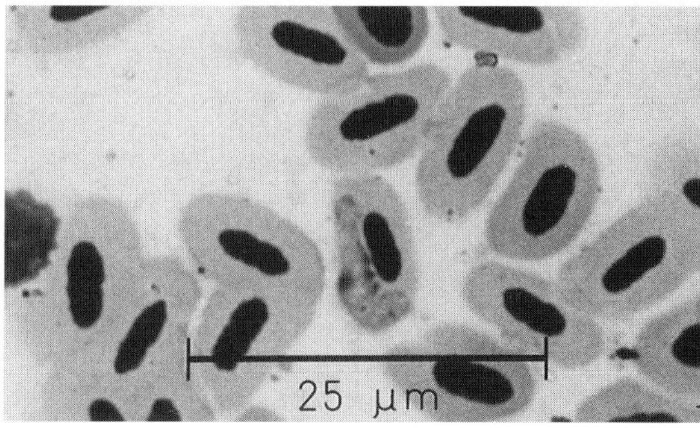

Figure 7.9 *P. (N.) vaughani* ex *Pycnonotus goiavier* (joint infection with *P. rouxi*), macrogametocyte; Kuala Kangsar, Malaysia, October 1959.

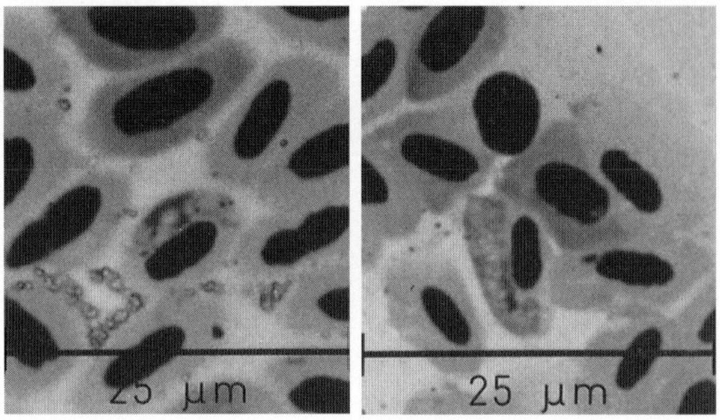

a b

Figure 7.10a *P. (N.) rouxi*, same slide as Figure 7.19, mature macrogametocyte.

Figure 7.10b *P. (N.) vaughani* ex *Pycnonotus goiavier* (joint infection with *P. (N.) rouxi*), same slide as Figure 7.9, macrogametocyte for size-comparison with that of the species in Figure 7.19.

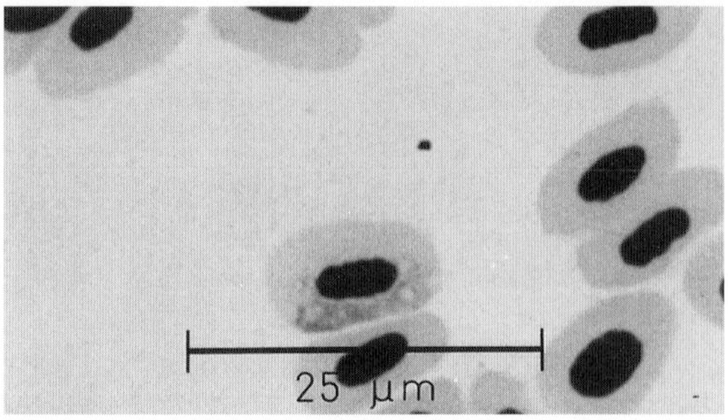

Figure 7.11 *P. (N.) vaughani* ex *Turdus obscurus*, gametocyte (stain faded); Mt Brinchang, Malaysia, 12 November 1961.

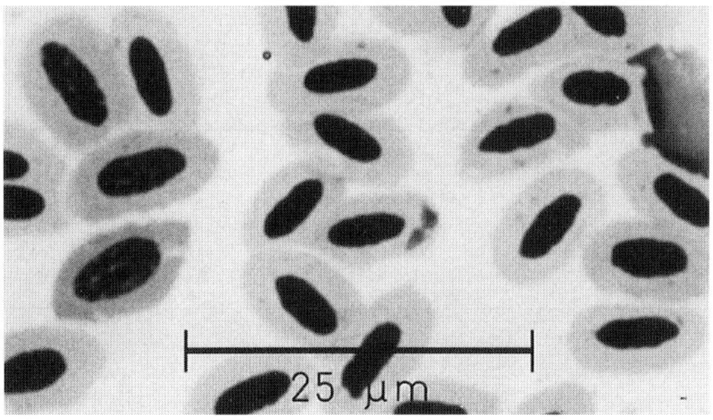

Figure 7.12 *P. (N.) rouxi* ex *Trichastoma rostratum* (joint infection with *P. (N.) corradettii* n.sp.), "bow-tie" schizont; Rantau Panjang, Malaysia, 6 September 1960.

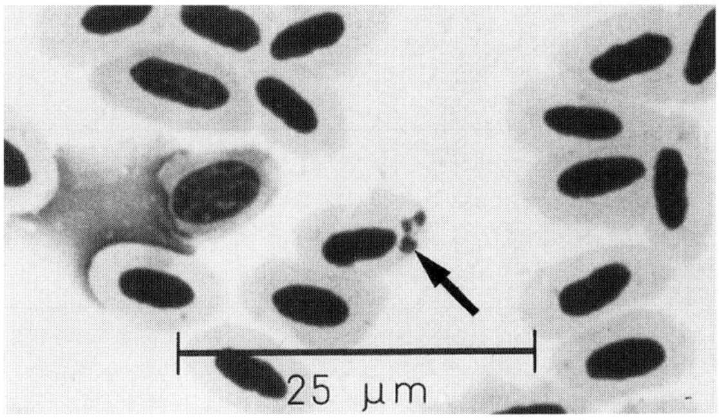

Figure 7.13 Same species and slide as Figure 7.12, one of the characteristic "bow-tie" elements divided, the other (arrowed) not so.

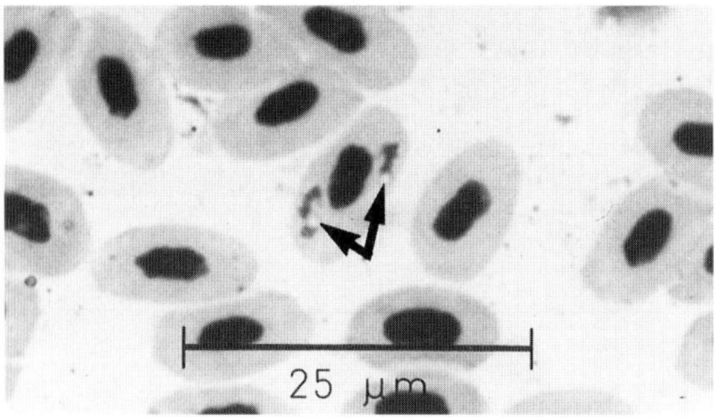

Figure 7.14 *P. (N.) rouxi* ex *Zoothera sibirica*, two schizonts (fan-shaped and linear) undergoing chromatin division in same erythrocyte, their vitreous globules arrowed; Mt Brinchang, Malaysia, 10 August 1962.

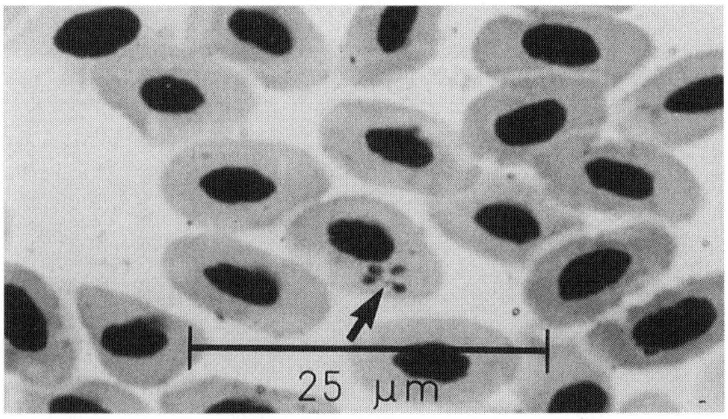

Figure 7.15 *P. (N.) rouxi* ex, same slide as Figure 7.14, cruciform schizont with tiny pigment dot arrowed (compare *P. vaughani*, Figure 7.4).

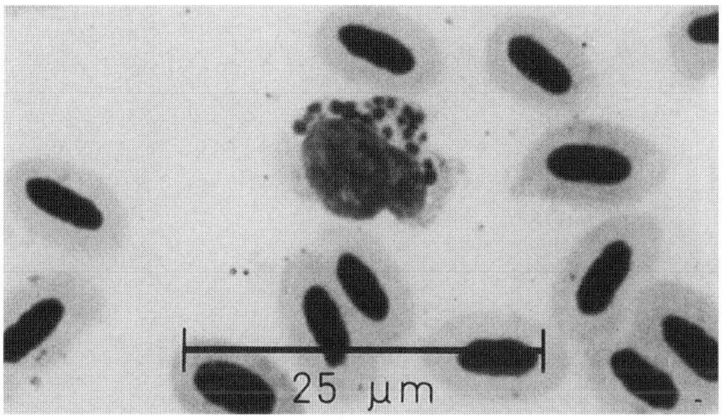

Figure 7.16 *P. (N.) rouxi* and *P. (N.) corradettii* n.sp., same slide as Figure 7.12, phagocytosed merozoites that could lead to confusion with *P. (Huffia) elongatum*.

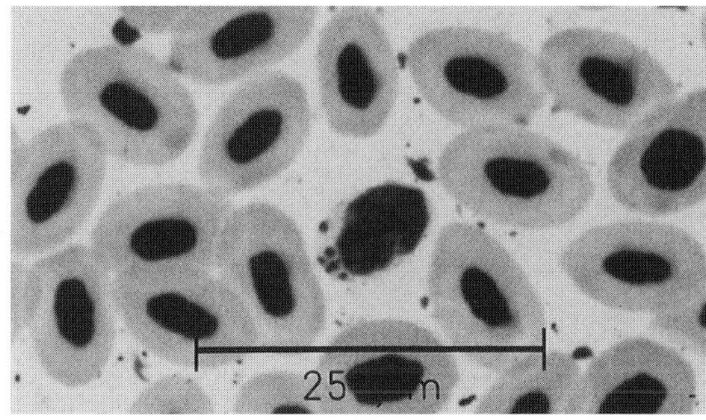

Figure 7.17 *P. (N.) rouxi* and *P. (N.) vaughani* ex *Zoothera sibirica*, six intraleucocytic merozoites which could easily be mistaken for an exoerythrocytic schizont of *P. (H.) elongatum*; Mt Brinchang, Malaysia, 14 December 1961.

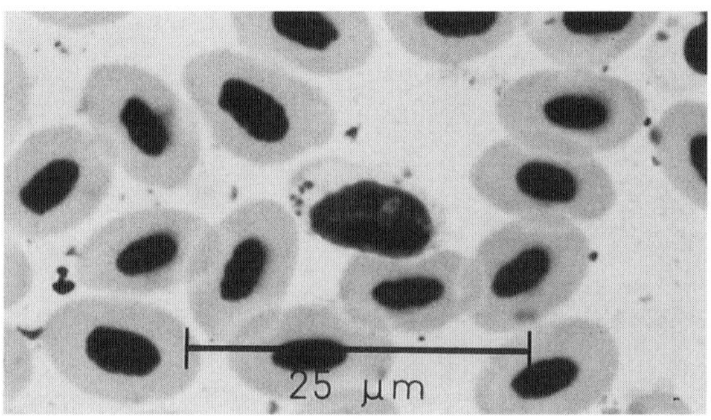

Figure 7.18 Same species and slide as Figure 7.17, phagocytosis clearly demonstrated by the diminished size of the intralymphocytic merozoites as compared with those of Figure 7.17.

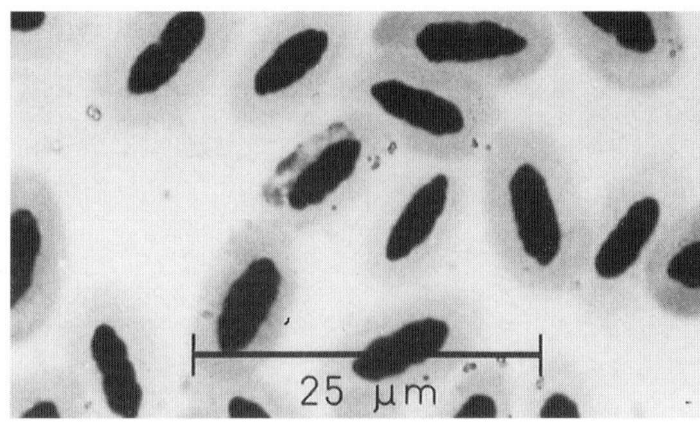

Figure 7.19 *P. (N.) rouxi* ex *Copsychus saularis* (joint infection with *P. (H.) matutinum*), same slide as Figure 5.11, mature microgametocyte.

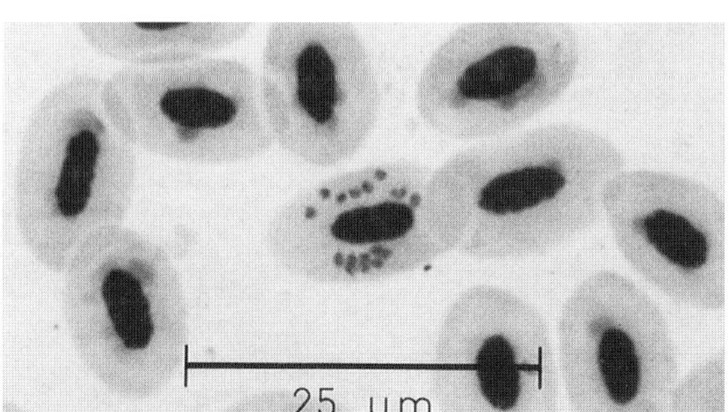

Figure 7.20 *P. (N.) nucleophilum* ex *Rallina eurizonoides*, two groups of eight fully condensed merozoites, the lowermost still retaining the shape of the segmenter and the other dispersed; Dalton Pass, Luzon, Philippines, 10 July 1960.

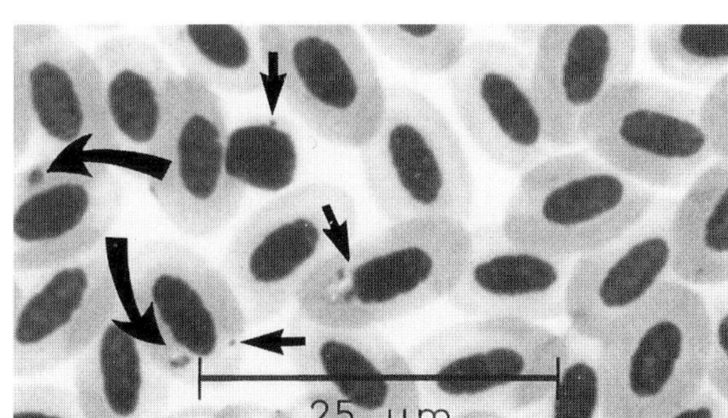

Figure 7.21 *P. (N.) nucleophilum* ex *Ploceus philippinus*, topmost straight arrow indicating an intralymphocytic merozoite, the lowermost one an intraerythrocytic example; for the remaining arrows see p. 78; Bang Phra, Cholburi, Thailand, 30 August 1966.

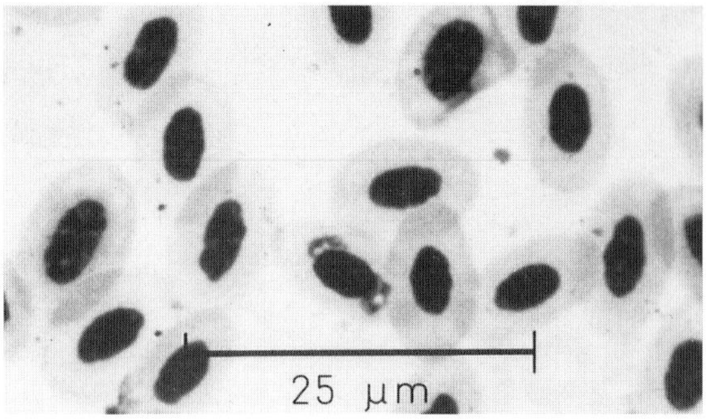

Figure 7.22 *P. (N.) nucleophilum*, same slide as Figures 7.3 and 7.24, doubly invaded erythrocyte with two polar schizonts.

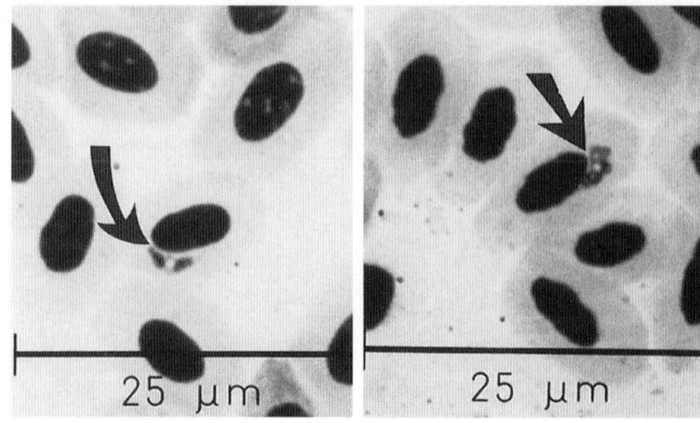

a b

Figure 7.23a *P. (N.) nucleophilum*, same slide as Figure 7.22, binucleate schizont arrowed to illustrate its having been pulled away from the host-cell nucleus through rapid drying at the thin edge of a blood smear.

Figure 7.23b *P. (N.) nucleophilum*, same slide as Figure 7.23(a) hexanucleate segmenter breaking free (arrow) from host-cell nucleus.

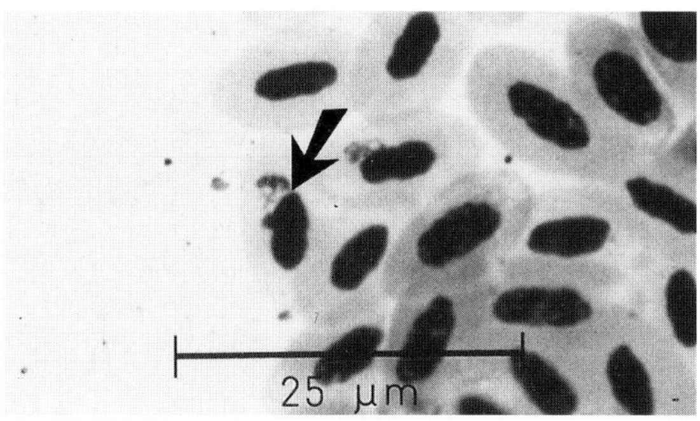

Figure 7.24 *P. (N.) nucleophilum*, same slide as Figure 7.3, tangential interface between vacuolated, quadrinucleate schizont and host-cell nucleus arrowed.

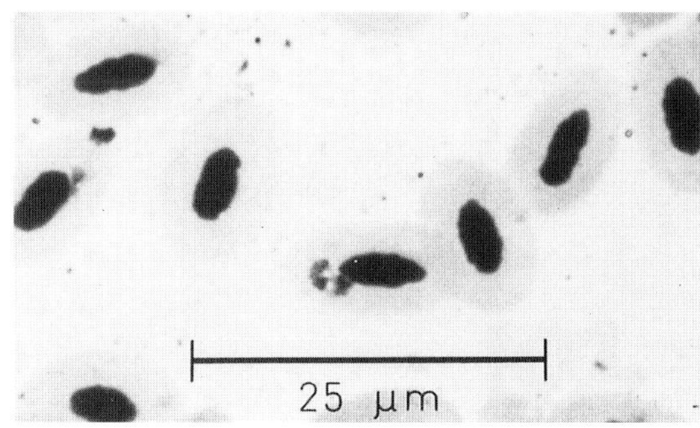

Figure 7.25 Same species and slide as Figure 7.3, quadrinucleate schizont with bright little vacuoles.

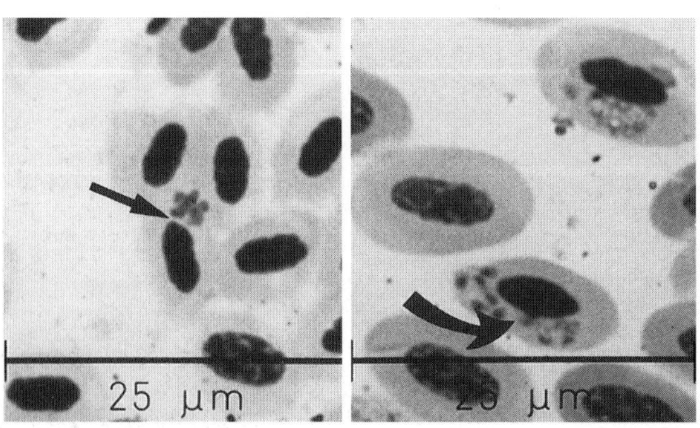

a b

Figure 7.26a *P. (N.) nucleophilum* ex *Nectarinia jugularis*, hexanucleate segmenter fully freed (arrow) from host-cell nucleus; Tarabanan, Palawan, Philippines, 13 May 1962.

Figure 7.26b *P. (N.) nucleophilum*, same slide as Figure 7.39, arrow indicating junction between two developing hexanucleate schizonts.

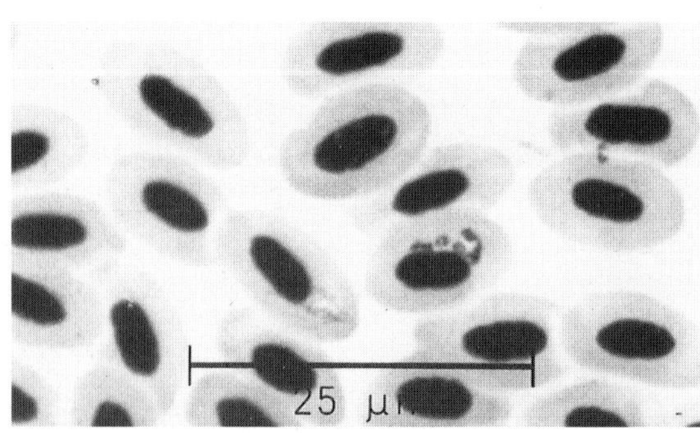

Figure 7.27 Same species and slide as Figure 7.21, octonucleate schizont resulting from final division of such a precursor as seen in Figure 7.3 (in which the four initial chromatin masses are particularly heavy).

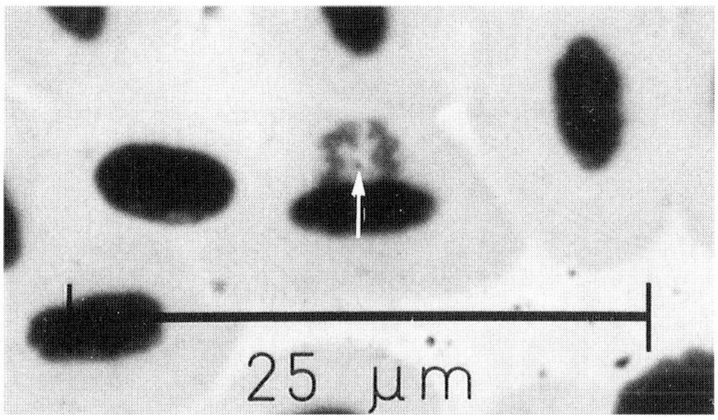

Figure 7.28 *P. (N.) nucleophilum* ex *Eudynamys scolopacea* (joint infection with *P. (H.) relictum* **s.l.**), nine-nucleate presegmenter, pigment dot arrowed; Palawan, Philippines, 15 May 1962.

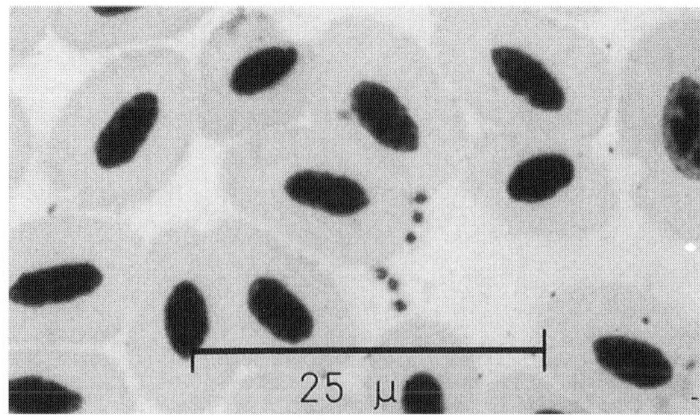

Figure 7.29 *P. (N.) nucleophilum* ex *Eudynamys scolopacea*, same slide as Figure 7.28, merozoite departure from host corpuscle.

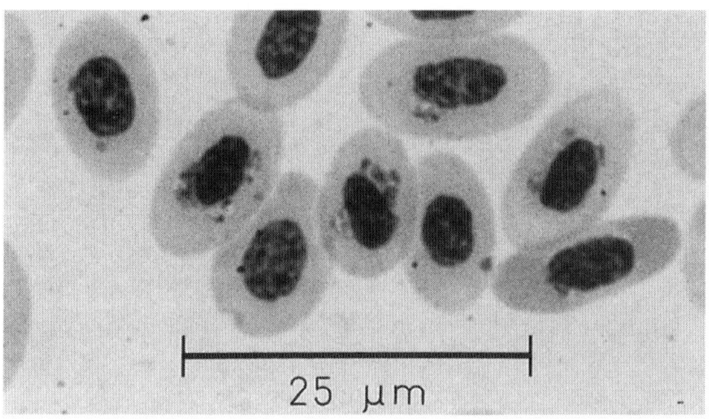

Figure 7.30 *P. (N.) nucleophilum* ex *Aplonis panayensis* (joint infection with *P. (H.) relictum* ssp. *relictum*), central erythrocyte with quadrinucleate schizont on right "shoulder" of nucleus, and early schizont to left; Puerto Princessa, Palawan, Philippines, 24 May 1962.

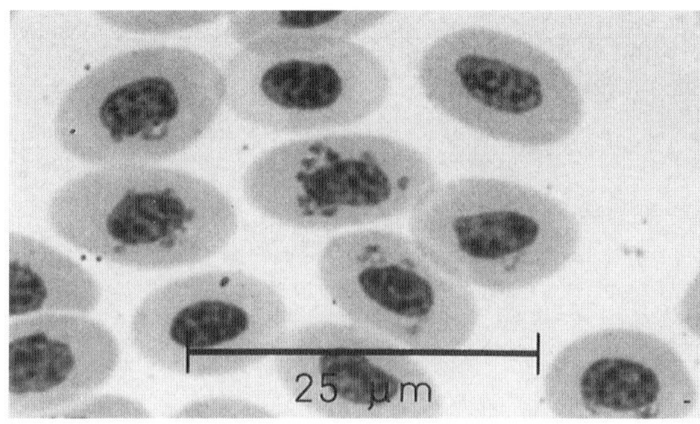

Figure 7.31 *P. (N.) nucleophilum* ex Red Junglefowl, uppermost schizont of top-central parasitized cell showing faint pigment at the tip of its extension towards right end of host-cell nucleus (compare Figure 7.30).

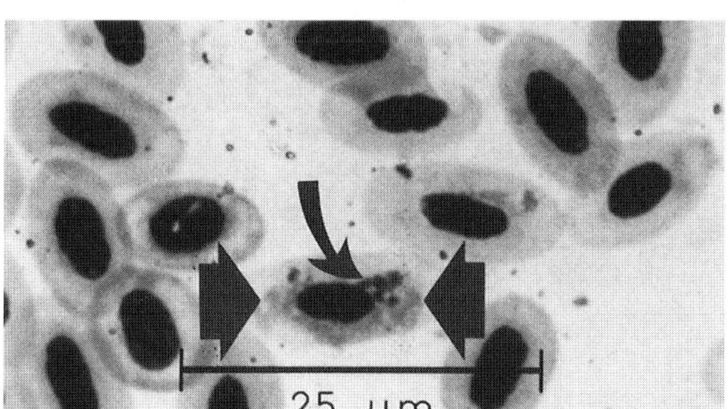

Figure 7.32 *P. (N.) nucleophilum* ex *Sturnus nigricollis*, same slide as Figure 7.3, double occupancy of red cell by hexanucleate schizont (arrowed) and *Haemoproteus pastoris*.

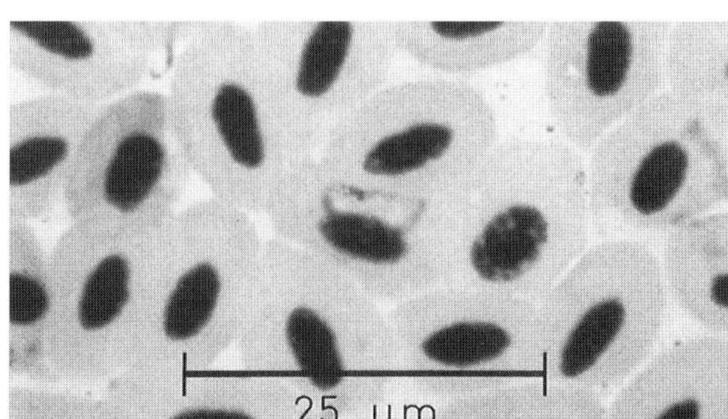

Figure 7.33 *P. (N.) nucleophilum* ex *Eudynamys scolopacea*, same slide as Figure 7.28, young microgametocyte with clumped pigment.

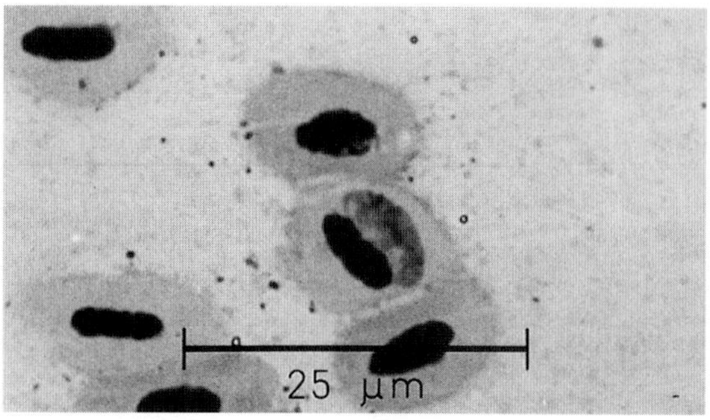

Figure 7.34 *P. (N.) nucleophilum* ex *Ixobrychus cinnamomeus*, macrogametocyte; Subang, Malaysia, 8 June 1962.

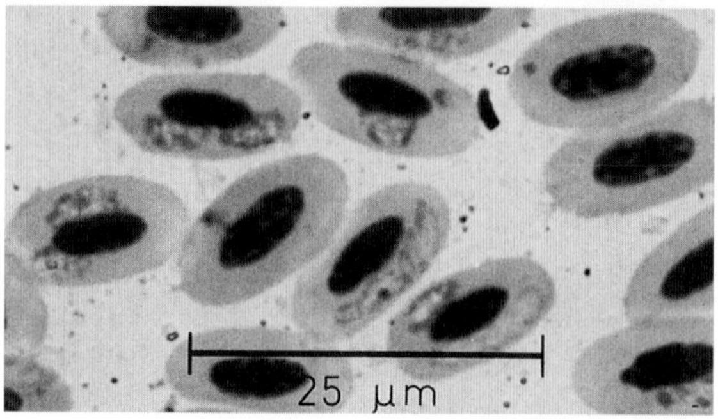

Figure 7.35 *P. (N.) nucleophilum* ex *Streptopelia chinensis*, same slide as Figure 7.26b, mature microgametocyte with clumped pigment.

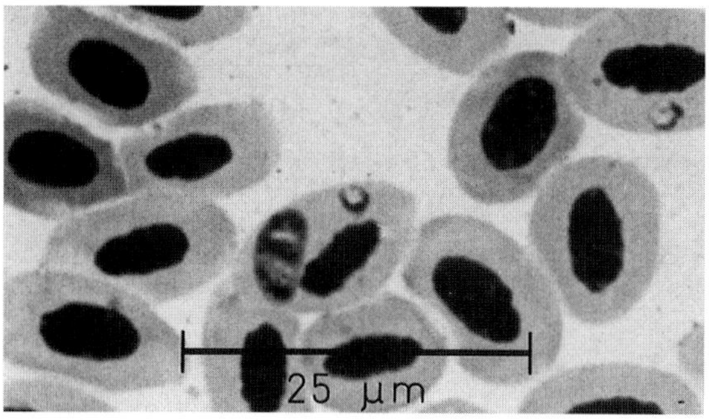

Figure 7.36 *P. (N.) corradettii* n.sp., same slide as Figure 3.1, signet-ring trophozoites with prominent vacuole in top-right and central erythrocytes, the latter also containing a mature macrogametocyte.

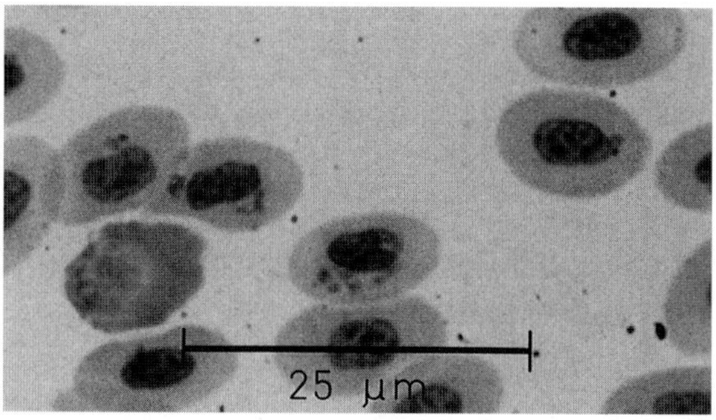

Figure 7.37 *P. (N.) nucleophilum* ex Red Junglefowl, same slide as Figure 5.6, with similar schizont to central one of Figure 7.30.

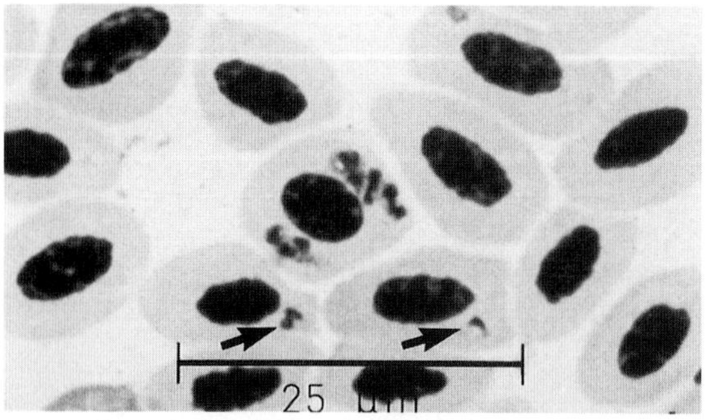

Figure 7.38 *P. (N.) corradettii* n.sp., same slide as Figure 3.1, erythrocyte to upper right of scale bar containing typical signet-ring trophozoite, its relatively heavy chromatin mass arrowed; that to its left with a schizont at the earliest division stage and with no cytoplasm apparent (arrowed); the hypertrophied red cell with a distorted nucleus above these, exhibiting three developing tri- to quadrinucleate schizonts.

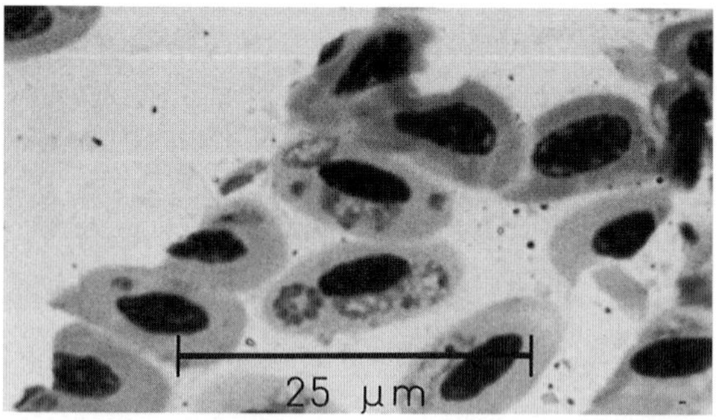

Figure 7.39 *P. (Novyella) corradettii* n.sp. (the rosette) and *P. (N.) nucleophilum* ex *Streptopelia chinensis*, both parasitized erythrocytes at centre showing slight lateral displacement of their nuclei; Siaton, Negros Oriental, Philippines, 17 February 1965.

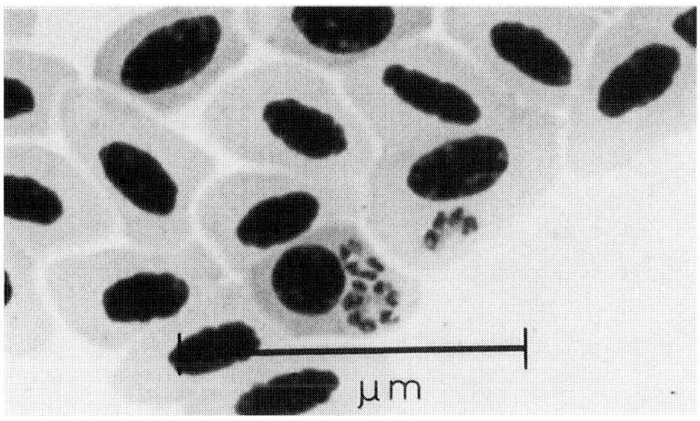

Figure 7.40 *P. (N.) corradettii* n.sp., same slide as Figure 7.36, nucleus of central red cell rounded up and displaced, the uppermost (quadrinucleate) schizont topped by a triangular pigment patch and the fan-shaped one to right enclosing a zone of fading pigment. The octonucleate rosette displays a similar zone.

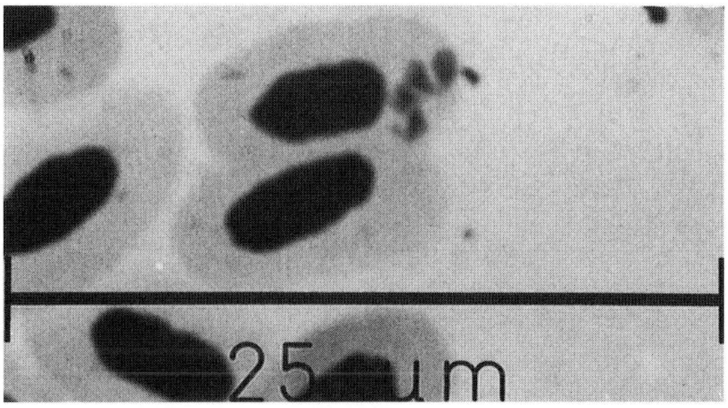

Figure 7.41 *P. (N.) corradettii* n.sp. ex *Trichastoma rostratum*, same slide as Figures 7.6a, 7.12 and 7.13, of *P. rouxi*, fan configuration of bulky separating merozoites showing pyriform shape prior to condensation.

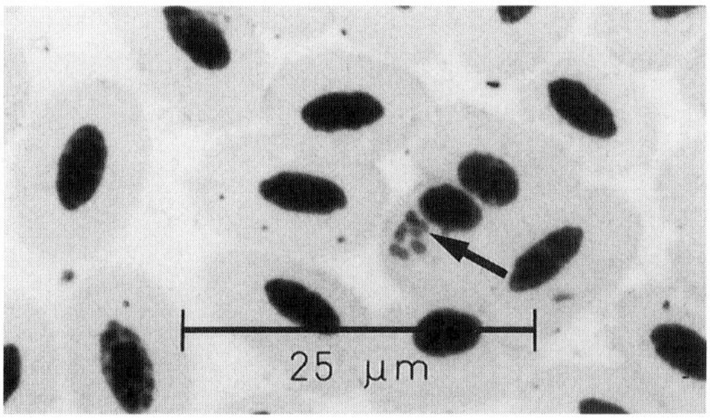

Figure 7.42 *P. (N.) corradettii* n.sp., same slide as Figure 7.39, six-merozoite segmenter with arrowed patch of brownish-golden pigment.

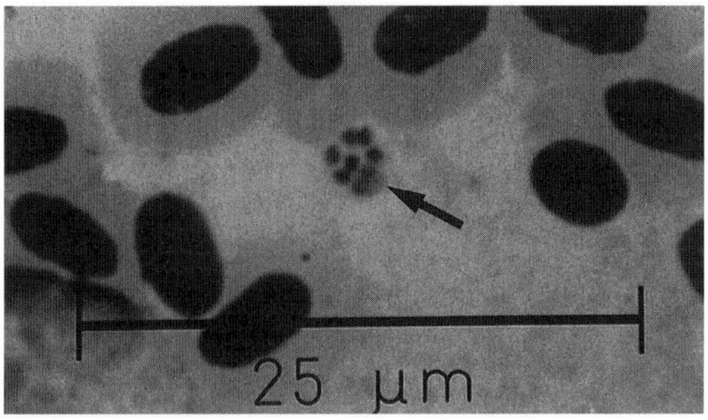

Figure 7.43 *P. (N.) corradettii* n.sp. ex *Nectarinia jugularis* (multiple infection with *P. (H.) matutinum* and *P. (N.) nucleophilum*), freed segmenter of six rounded-up merozoites with relatively huge patch of brownish-golden pigment arrowed; Tarabanan, Palawan, Philippines, 13 May 1962.

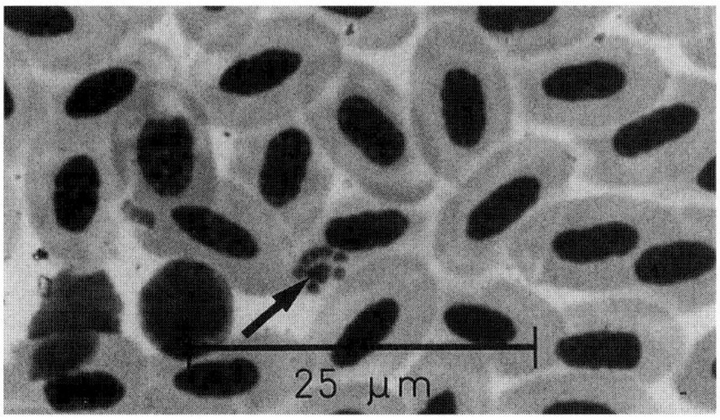

Figure 7.44 *P. (N.) corradettii* n.sp. ex *Chalcophaps indica* (multiple infection with *P. (H.) matutinum* and *P. (N.) nucleophilum*), eight-merozoite segmenter with characteristically dominating pigment patch arrowed near centre of open rosette; Tarabanan, Palawan, Philippines, 13 May 1962.

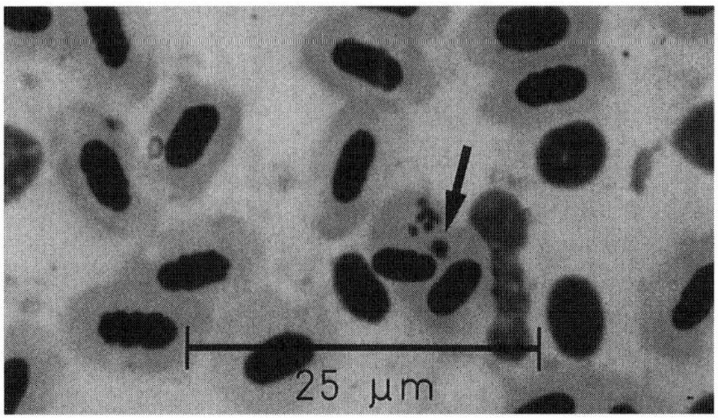

Figure 7.45 *P. (N.) corradettii* n.sp., same slide as Figure 7.43, six-merozoite segmenter, the large brownish-golden pigment patch arrowed.

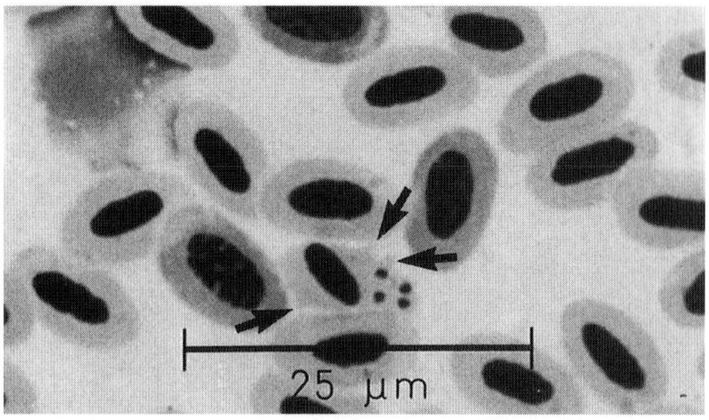

Figure 7.46 *P. (N.) corradettii* n.sp., same slide as Figure 7.12, four merozoites dispersed in an erythrocyte with tilted and displaced nucleus and cell membrane drawn out into (arrowed) points.

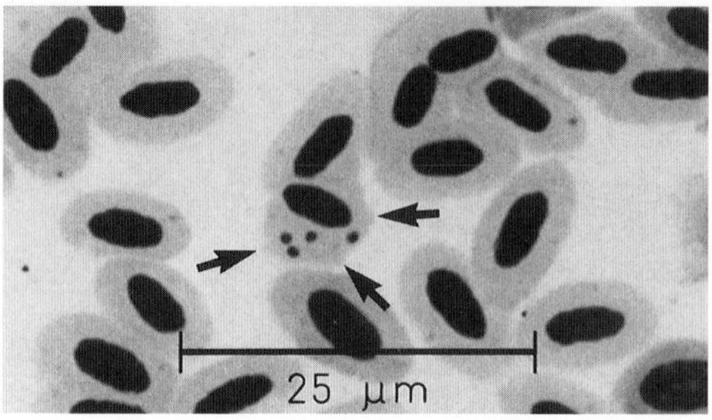

Figure 7.47 *P. (N.) corradettii* n.sp., same slide as Figure 7.46; a further example of displacement of the nucleus of the parasitized corpuscle and fimbriation of its membrane (points arrowed) prior to departure of merozoites.

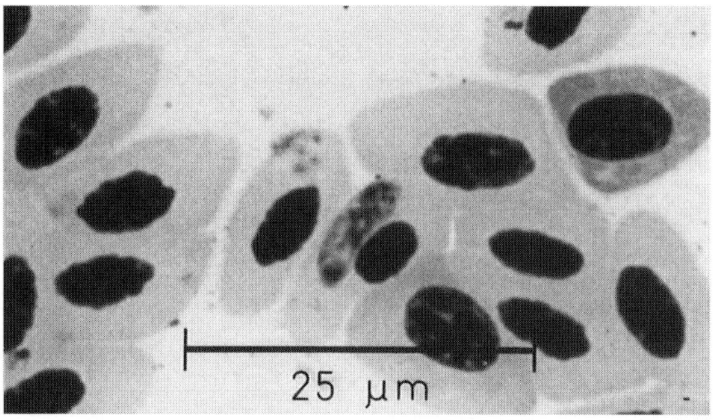

Figure 7.48 *P. (N.) corradettii* n.sp., same slide as Figure 7.49, microgametocyte alongside laterally displaced, shrunken and ovoidal host-cell nucleus.

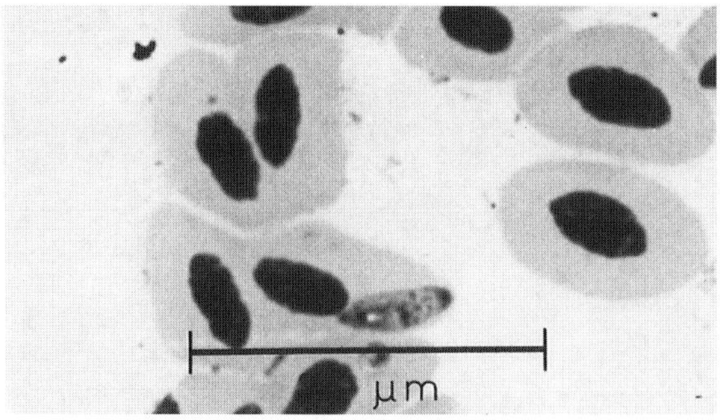

Figure 7.49 *P. (N.) corradettii* n.sp., same slide as Figure 3.1; polar microgametocyte, host-cell nucleus displaced laterally and to the opposite pole.

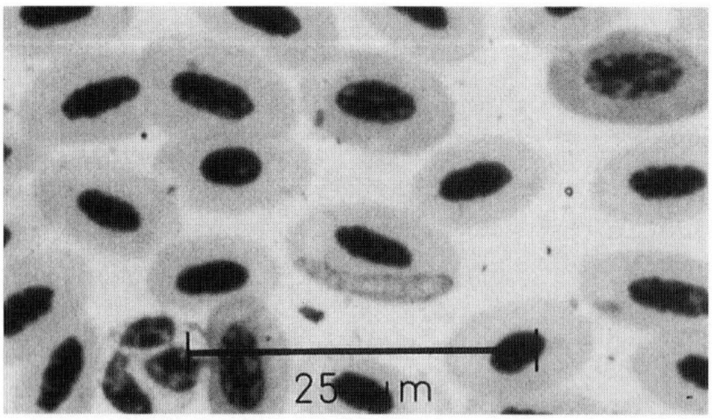

Figure 8.1 *P. (Huffia) elongatum* ex *Trichastoma elongatum* (multiple infection with *P. (H.) matutinum* and *P. (G.) dissanaikei*), exhibiting Garnham's (1966) "thin emaciated aspect" and being "strikingly elongate in shape" and in a "somewhat hypertrophied" host-cell with its nucleus only slightly displaced laterally; Rantau Panjang, Malaysia, 8 March 1960.

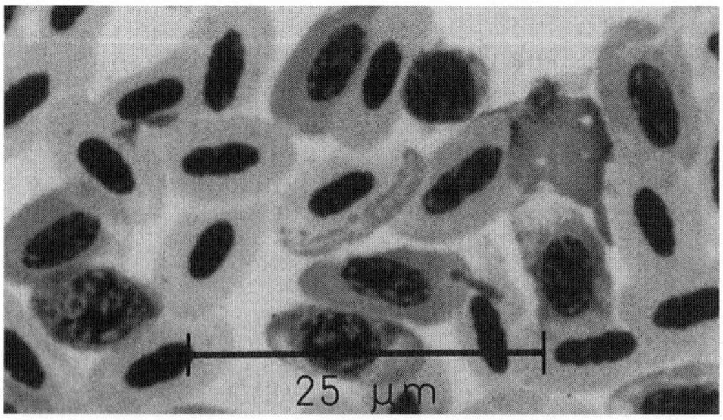

Figure 8.2 *P. (Huffia) elongatum*, same slide as Figure 8.1, showing the gap between gametocyte and host-cell nucleus and the former's opposite margin closely appressed to the cell membrane as in figure 8, plate LVIII of Garnham (1966).

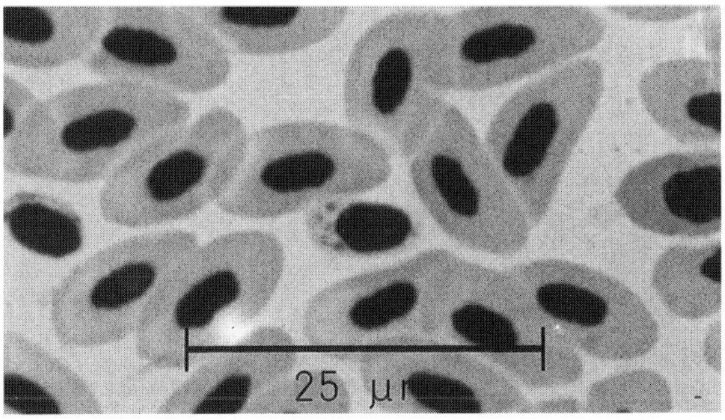

Figure 8.3 *P. (Huffia) elongatum* ex *Pachycephala grisola*, immature exoerythrocytic schizont; Mt Brinchang, Malaysia, 10 February 1959.

References

Adene, D. F. and Dipeolu, O. O., Survey of blood and ectoparasites of domestic fowls in Ibadan, Western State of Nigeria, *Bull. Anim. Health Prod. Afr.* **23**, 333–335 (1981).

Africa, C. M., Dy, F. J. and Soriano, L. J., A study on the identity of a *Plasmodium* in the Philippine domestic fowl (*Gallus gallus*), *Univ. Philipp. Nat. Appl. Sci. Bull.* **7**, 279–289 (1940).

Akiba, K. [Studies on avian malaria. II. On the species of *Plasmodium* from the chicken in Japan (*P. japonicum* Ishiguro, 1957) a synonym for *P. juxtanucleare* Versiani and Gomes, 1941], *Jpn J. Vet. Sci.* **21**, 18 (1959). *In Japanese.*

Al-Dabagh, M. A., The incidence of blood parasites in wild and domestic birds of Columbus, Ohio, *Am. Midl. Nat.* **72**, 148–151 (1964).

Ashford, R. S., Palmer, T. T., Ash, J. S. and Bray, R. S., Blood parasites of Ethiopian birds. 1. General survey, *J. Wildl. Dis.* **12**, 409–426 (1976).

Austin, O. L., Jr, *Birds of the World.* New York: Golden Press, 1961.

Ayala, S. C. and Varela, C. E., Malaria in *Chordeiles minor* (Aves: Caprimulgidae), an intercontinental migrant, *Rev. Inst. Med. Trop. Sao Paulo* **17**, 253–256 (1975).

Basu, B. C., Studies on a malaria infection in a paddy bird, *J. Malar. Inst. India* **1**, 273–284 (1938).

Bauer, O. N., Parazitofauna nekotorykh ptits Zakavkaz'ya, sovershayushchikh vertikal'nye migratsii [Parasite fauna of some birds from Transcaucasia, which undertake vertical migrations], *Uch. zap. Leningr. ordena Lenina gos. univ. im. A. A. Zhdanova, Ser. biol. nauk* **11**, 77–91 (1939).

Bauer, O. N., Parazitofauna ptits vysokogornoi chasti Borzhomskogo raiona [Parasite fauna of birds from the high-mountain part of the Borzhomskii region], *Uch. zap. Leningr. ordena Lenina gos. univ. im. A. A. Zhdanova, Ser. biol. nauk* **18**, 63–92 (1941).

Bennett, G. F., Bishop, M. A. and Peirce, M. A., The species and distribution of the haemoproteids of the avian family Muscicapidae *sensu lato* (Passeriformes), *J. Nat. History* **25**, 23–43 (1991).

Bennett, G. F., Blancou, J., White, E. M. and Williams, N. A., Blood parasites of some birds from Senegal. *J. Wildl. Dis.* **14**, 67–73 (1978).

Bennett, G. F. and Campbell, A. G., Avian Haemoproteidae, I. Description of *Haemoproteus fallisi* n.sp. and a review of the haemoproteids of the family Turdidae, *Can. J. Zool.* **50**, 1269–1275 (1972).

Bennett, G. F., Earlé, R. A., du Toit, H. and Huchzermeyer, F. W., A host-parasite catalogue of the haematozoa of the sub-Saharan birds, *Onderstepoort J. vet. Res* **59**, 1–73 (1992).

Bennett, G. F., Eyles, D. E., Warren, McW. and Cheong, W. H., *Plasmodium juxtanucleare* (?) a newly discovered parasite of domestic fowl in Malaya, *Singapore Med. J.* **4**, 172–173 (1963).

Bennett, G. F. and Laird, M., The work of the World Health Organization International Reference Centre for Avian Malaria Parasites in 1969 (WHO/MAL 70.712, 5 pp. Mimeograph, Geneva, 1970), *WHO Chronicle* **25**, 17–19 (1971).

Bennett, G. F., Okia, N. O. and Cameron, M. F., Avian hematozoa of some Ugandan birds, *J. Wildl. Dis.* **10**, 458–465 (1974).

Bennett, G. F. and Peirce, M. A., The haemoproteids of the avian family Phasianidae, *Can J. Zool.* **67**, 1557–1565 (1989).

Bennett, G. F. and Peirce, M. A., The haemoproteids of the weaver finches (Passeriformes), *J. Nat. History* **25**, 7–22 (1991).

Bennett, G. F., Peirce, M. A. and Caines, J. R., Avian Haemoproteidae, 19. The haemoproteids of the sunbirds (family Nectariniidae) and morphometric variation in *Haemoproteus sequeirae, Can. J. Zool.* **63**, 1371–1376 (1984).

Bennett, G. F., Whiteway, M. and Woodworth-Lynas, C. B., *A Host-Parasite Catalogue of the Avian Haematozoa*, Occ. Pprs in Biol. No. 5. St John's, Newfoundland, Memorial University of Newfoundland, 1982.

Berger, A. J., *Hawaiian Birdlife*. Honolulu: The University Press of Hawaii, 1972.

Bishop, M. A. and Bennett, G. F., The haemoproteids of the avian order Strigiformes, *Can. J. Zool.* **67**, 2676–2684 (1989).

Bishop, M. A. and Bennett, G. F., The haemoproteids of the avian families Corvidae (crows and jays) and Sturnidae (starlings and mynas) (Passeriformes), *Can. J. Zool.* **68**, 2251–2256 (1990).

Bisseru, B. and Lim, K. C., Parasitic fauna (faeces and blood) of the "Klang" house crow, *Corvus splendens protegatus, Southeast Asian J. Trop. Med. Publ. Hlth* **2**, 412 (1971).

Bray, R. S., VI. *Laverania falciparum. Am. J. Trop. Med. Hyg.* **7**, 20–24 (1958).

Bray, R. S., Classification of the avian malaria parasites, *Trans. R. Soc. Trop. Med. Hyg.* **57**, 229 (1963).

Brumpt, E., Paludisme aviaire: *Plasmodium gallinaceum* n.sp. de la poule domestique, *C. R. hebd. Séanc. Acad. Sci. Paris* **200**, 783–786 (1935).

Burtikashvili, L. P., Kroveparazity vorob'inykh ptits Gruzii [Blood parasites of passeriform birds from Georgia], *Materialy Pervogo s~btezda Vsesoyuz. obshch. protozoologov. Baku* 19–21 (1971).

Burtikashvili, L. P., Parazyti krovi dikikh ptits Gruzii [Blood parasites of wild birds in Georgia], *Metsniereba, Tbilisi* 1–123 (1978).

Cassamagnagli, A., Plasmodiosis (malario o paludismo) en las aves del Uruguay, *Third Cong. Bras. Vet.* 625–628 (1945a).

Cassamagnagli, A., Enfermedades parasitarias causades por hematozoarios en las aves del Uruguay, *Third Cong. Bras. Vet.* (1945b), pp. 645–660.

Cassamagnagli, A., Malaria en las aves del Uruguay, *Bol. Mens. Dir. Ganad. (Montevideo)* **29**, 105–129 (1944a).

Cassamagnagli, A., Malaria en las aves del Uruguay, *Fac. de Vet. (Montevideo).* 1947b, 93 pp.

Coggeshall, L. T., *Plasmodium lophurae*, a new species of malaria parasite pathogenic for the domestic fowl, *Am. J. Hyg.* **27**, 615–618 (1938).

Corradetti, A., Garnham, P. C. C. and Laird, M., New classification of the avian malaria parasites. *Parassitol.* **5**, 1–4 (1963).

Corradetti, A. and Scanga, M., Segnalazione in Europa di *Plasmodium (Giovannolaia) polare* Manwell, 1934 nel nuovo ospite *Falco tinnunculus* e studi sulla biologia di questo plasmodio, *Parassitol.* **5**, 19–27 (1963).

Corradetti, A. and Scanga, M., Notes on *Plasmodium (Giovannolaia) polare* and its transmission with *Culiseta longiareolata*, Parassitol. **7**, 61–64 (1965).

Corradetti, A. and Scanga, M., *Plasmodium (Novyella) vaughani* subsp. *merulae*, n.subsp., parassita di *Turdus merula* con descriziona del ciclo pre-eritrocitio, *Parassitol.* **14**, 85–93 (1972).

Corradetti, A. and Scanga, M., The *Plasmodium vaughani* complex, *Exp. Parasitol.* **34**, 344–349 (1973).

Corradetti, A. Garnham, P. C. C., Neri, I., Scanga, M. and Cavallini, C., A redescription of *Plasmodium (Haemamoeba) relictum* (Grassi and Feletti, 1891), *Parassitol.* **12**, 1–12 (1970).

Corradetti, A., Neri, I., Palmieri, C., Verolini, F., Giulani, V. and Scanga, M., Note su *Plasmodium vaughani* e su un plasmodio con ciclo schizogonico endo-emoblastico di tipo *elongatum* rinvenuti in *Turdus merula, Parassitol.* **3**, 97–100 (1961).

Corradetti, A., Neri, I. and Scanga, M., Segnalazione in Italia di *Plasmodium praecox* var. *matutinum in Turdus iliacus*, a separazione di questo plasmodio da *Plasmodium praecox* come specie distinta: *Plasmodium matutinum* Huff, 1937, *Parassitol.* **2**, 333–343 (1960).

Corradetti, A., Verolini, F. and Neri, I., *Plasmodium (Haemamoeba) giovannolai n.sp. parassita di Turdus merula, Parassitol.* **5**, 11–18 (1963).

Crawford, R. D., Domestic fowl, in *Evolution of Domesticated Animals*, ed. I. L. Mason. London-New York: Longman, 1984, pp. 298–311.

Danilewsky, B., On the parasites of the blood (Haematozoa), *Russ. Med.* **9**, 46–48 (1884). *In Russian.*

Danilewsky, B. *La Parasitologie Comparée du Sang*. I. Nouvelles recherches sur les parasites du sang des oiseaux. Kharkov, 1889.

Darlington, P. J., Jr, *Zoogeography: The Geographical Distribution of Animals*. New York: Ronald Press, 1957.

de Jong, A. D., *Plasmodium dissanaikei* n.sp. a new avian malaria parasite from the rose-ringed parakeet of Ceylon, *Psittacula krameri manillensis, Ceylon J. Med. Sci.* **20**, 41–45 (1971).

de Mello, I. F., Further contributions to the study of the blood parasites of the Indian birds, together with a list of the hemoparasites hitherto recorded, *J. Asiatic Soc. Bengal, Sci.*, **II**, 95–122 (1936).

Delacour, J., *The Pheasants of the World*. London: Country Life, 1965.

Dhanapala, S. B., The occurrence of *Plasmodium juxtanucleare* Versiani and Gomes 1941 in domestic fowls in Ceylon, *Riv. Malariol.* **41**, 39–46 (1962).

Dissanaike, A. S., On some blood parasites of wild animals in Ceylon, *Ceylon Vet. J.* **11**, 75–86 (1963).

Earlé, R. A., Huchzermeyer, F. W., Bennett, G. F. and Little, R. M., Occurrence of *Plasmodium juxtanucleare* in greywing francolin, *South African Journal of Wildlife Research*, **21**, 30–32 (1991).

Edwards, E. P., *A Coded List of Birds of the World*. Sweet Briar, Virginia: Ernest P. Edwards, 1974.

Fernando, M. A. and Dissanaike, A. S., Malaria parasites of the Malayan jungle fowl *Gallus gallus spadiceus, Southeast Asian J. Trop. Med. Publ. Hlth.* **5**, 144 (1974).

Fernando, M. A. and Dissanaike, A. S., Studies on *Plasmodium gallinaceum* and *Plasmodium juxtanucleare* from the Malayan jungle fowl *Gallus gallus spadiceus, Southeast Asian J. Trop. Med. Publ. Hlth.* **6**, 25–32 (1975).

Gabaldon, A. and Ulloa, G., A new species of the subgenus *Novyella* (Haemosporina, Plasmodidae) from *Aramides cajanea* (Gruiformes, Rallidae), in *Parasitological Topics*, ed. E. U. Canning. Lawrence, Kansas: Society of Protozoologists, 1981, pp. 100–105.

Garnham, P. C. C., Terminology of Haemosporidiidea, in *5th Int. Congr. Trop. Med. Malar.*, Vol. 2, Istanbul. 1953, pp. 228–231.

Garnham, P. C. C., The subgenera of *Plasmodium* in mammals, *Annls. Soc. belge Méd. Trop.* **44**, 267–272 (1964).

Garnham, P. C. C., *Malaria Parasites and Other Haemosporidia*. Oxford: Blackwell Scientific Publications, 1966.

Garnham, P. C. C., Bird, R. G. and Baker, J. R., Electron microscope studies of motile stages of malaria parasites; III. The ookinetes of *Haemamoeba* and *Plasmodium, Trans. R. Soc. Trop. Med. Hyg.* **56**, 116–120 (1962).

Garnham, P. C. C. and Duggan, A. J., *Catalogue of the Garnham Collection of Malaria Parasites and Other Haemosporidia*. London: The Wellcome Trust, 1986.

Gaud, J. and Petitot, M. L., Hématozoaires des oiseaux du Maroc, *Arch. Inst. Pasteur Maroc* **3**, 149–171 (1945).

Giovannola, A., I plasmodi aviari, *Riv. Parassit.* **3**, 221–266 (1939).

Glushchenko, V. V., Materialy do vivchennya sezonnoi dinamiki krovoparazitiv ptakhiv u Kiivs'komu polissi [An investigation of the seasonal dynamics of blood parasites of birds from the Kiev forest], *Zb. pr. Zool. muz. Akad. nauk. Ukr. SSR* **31**, 56–62 (1962).

Glushchenko, V. V., Parazitofauna krovi domashnikh i dikikh ptits Kievskogo Poles'ya [Blood parasite fauna of domestic and wild birds from the Kievskoe Poles'e Region], *Avtoreferat Dissertatsii, Inst. Zool. AN Ukr. SSR, Kiev.* 1963, 18 pp.

Golgi, C., Sul infezione malarica, *J. R. Accad. Med. Torino* **33**, 734–783 (1885).

Golgi, C., Sul ciclo evolutivo dei parassiti malarici nella febre terzana; diagnosi differenziale tra i parassiti endoglobulari malarici della terzana et quelli della quartana, *Archs. Sc. méd.* **13**, 173–195 (1889).

Grassi, B., Studi di uno zoologo sulla malaria, *Mem. Rend. Accad. dei Lincei* **53**, 299–302 (1900).

Grassi, B. and Feletti, R., Parasites malariques chez les oiseaux, *Archo. ital. Biol.* **13**, 297–300 (1890).

Grassi, B. and Feletti, R., Nuova contribuzione allo studio della malaria, *Buoll. mens. Acad. Gioenia. Sci. nat. Catania* **16**, 16–20 (1891).

Grassi, B. and Feletti, R., Contribuzione allo studio dei parassiti malarici, *Atti Accad. gioenia Sci. nat. Catania*, Memoir **5**, 1–80 (1892).

Gray, A. P., *Bird Hybrids*. Farnham Royal, Bucks, England, Commonwealth Agricultural Bureaux, 1958.

Greiner, E. C. and Mundy, P. J., Hematozoa from southern African vultures, with a description of *Haemoproteus janovyi* sp.n, *J. Parasitol.* **65**, 147–153 (1979).

Greiner, E. C., Bennett, G. F., Laird, M. and Herman, C. M., Avian haematozoa. 2. Taxonomic keys and color pictorial guide to species of *Plasmodium*. *Wildl. Dis.* 75–3 (1975). *Forty-four coloured photomicrographs on microfiche No. 68.*

Greiner, E. C., Black, D. J. and Iverson, W. O., *Plasmodium* in a bald eagle (*Haliaeetus leucocephalus*) in Florida, *J. Wildl. Dis.* **17**, 555–558 (1981).

Haiba, M. H., Plasmodia of common Egyptian birds, *J. Comp. Path. Ther.* **58**, 207–210 (1948).

Hamerton, A. E., Report on the deaths occurring in the Society's Gardens during the year 1928, *Proc. Zool. Soc. Lond.* 49–59 (1929).

Hamerton, A. E., Report on the deaths occurring in the Society's Gardens during the year 1933, *Proc. Zool. Soc. Lond.* 389–442 (1934).

Hartman, E., Three species of bird malaria, *Plasmodium praecox, Plasmodium cathemerium* n.sp and *Plasmodium inconstans* n.sp., *Arch. Protinstenkd.* **60**, 1–7 (1927).

Hewitt, R., *Bird Malaria*. Baltimore: The Johns Hopkins Press, 1940.

Hewitt, R., Studies on the host parasite relationships of untreated infections with *Plasmodium lophurae* in ducks, *Am. J. Hyg.* **36**, 6–42 (1942).

Ho, Ping-ti, The indigenous origins of Chinese agriculture, in *Origins of Agriculture*, (ed. C. A. Reed). The Hague, Paris: Mouton Publishers, 1977, pp. 413–484.

Huchzermeyer, F. W., A host-parasite list of the haematozoa of domestic poultry in sub-Saharan Africa and the isolation of *Plasmodium durae* Herman from turkeys and francolins in South Africa, *Onderstepoort J. Vet. Res.* **60**, 15–21 (1993).

Huff, C. G., *Plasmodium elongatum* n.sp., an avian malarial organism with an elongate gametocyte, *Am. J. Hyg.* **11**, 385–391 (1930).

Huff, C. G., *Plasmodium hexamerium* n.sp. from the bluebird inoculable to canaries, *Am. J. Hyg.* **22**, 274–277 (1935).

Huff, C. G., A new variety of *Plasmodium relictum* from the robin, *J. Parasitol.* **23**, 400–404 (1937).

Huff, C. G., A survey of blood parasites of birds caught for banding purposes, *J. Amer. Vet. Assoc.* **90**, 615–620 (1939).

Huff, C. G., Coulston, F., Laird, R. L. and Porter, A. J., Pre-erythrocytic development of *Plasmodium lophurae* in various hosts, *J. Infect. Dis.* **81**, 7–13 (1947).

Huff, C. G., Pipkin, A. C., Weathersby, A. B. and Jensen, D. V., The morphology and behaviour of living exoerythrocytic stages of *Plasmodium gallinaceum* and *P. fallax* and their host cells, *J Biophys. Biochem. Cytol.* **7**, 93–102 (1960).

International Code of Zoological Nomenclature, 3rd ed. London: International Trust for Zoological Nomenclature, 1985.

Ishiguro, H., [Studies of domestic fowl malaria. I. A new species of malaria parasite, pathogenic to domestic fowl and its pathogenicity and transmission], *Jpn J. Vet. Sci.* **19**, 32–33, 129 (1957a). *In Japanese.*

Ishiguro, H., [*Plasmodium japonicum*, a new species of malaria parasite pathogenic for the domestic fowl], *Bull. Fac. Agr. Yamaguti Univ.* **8**, 723–733 (1957b). *In Japanese.*

Jones, W. H. S., *Malaria: A Neglected Factor in the History of Greece and Rome.* Cambridge: MacMillan & Bowes, 1907.

Kairullaev, K. K., Kroveparazit dikikh ptits poym crednego techeniya r. Urala [Blood parasites of wild birds in the floodplain of the middle Ural River in Kazakh SSR], *Izv. Akad. nauk Kaz. SSR Ser. Biol.* **17**, 19–21 (1979).

Kano, R., [Studies on bird malaria (5). Description of blood parasites in Japanese wild birds with remarks on unrecorded species], *Nippon Saikingaku Zasshi* **5**, 107–111 (1950). *In Japanese.*

King, A. F. A., Insects and disease. Mosquitoes and malaria. *Popular Science Monthly (NY)* **23**, 644–658 (1883).

King, B. F. and Dickinson, E. C., *A Field Guide to the Birds of South-east Asia*, Boston: Houghton Mifflin, 1975.

Kucera, J., Krevni parazite nasich ptaku se zvlastnim zretelem na krevny prvoki, [Blood parasites of our birds with special reference to the haemoprotozoa]. Thesis, Faculty of Natural Sciences, Charles University, Prague, Czechoslovakia 1978, 180 pp.

Laird, M., *Plasmodium vaughani* Novy and MacNeal, 1904, in the New Hebrides: with a note on the occurrence of *elongatum*-type exoerythrocytic schizogony in this species, *J. Parasitol.* **39**, 357–364 (1953).

Laird, M., Malayan Protozoa 5. Two avian malaria parasites, *J. Protozool.* **9**, 21–26 (1962).

Laird, M., The species of *Plasmodium* parasitizing birds in Malaysia, In *Proc. First Int. Cong. Parasitol.*, Vol. 1, Rome, 1964. Oxford: Pergamon Press 1966, pp. 234–235.

Laird, M., *Plasmodium durae* Herman from the introduced common peafowl in northern Nigeria, *J. Protozool.* **25**, 21–24 (1978).

Laird, M. and Bennett, G. F., The subarctic epizootiology of *Leucocytozoon simondi*, *J. Parasitol.* **56** Sec. 2, 198 (1970).

Laird, M. and Grewal, M. S., Avian malaria in the Oriental and Australian Regions, in *Eighth Int. Cong. Trop. Med. Malar.*, Teheran, 1968. pp. 1267–1268.

Laird, M. and Lari, F. A., Observations on *Plasmodium circumflexum* Kikuth and *P. vaughani* Novy and MacNeal from East Pakistan, *J. Parasitol.* **44**, 136–152 (1958).

Laird, M. and van Riper, C., III, Questionable reports of *Plasmodium* from birds in Hawaii, with the recognition of *P. relictum ssp. capistranoae* (Russell, 1932) as the avian malaria parasite there, in *Parasitological Topics*, ed. E. U. Canning. Lawrence, Kansas: Society of Protozoologists, 1981, pp. 159–165.

Laveran, A., Note sur un nouveau parasite trouvé dans le sang de plusieurs malades atteints de fièvre palustre, *Bull. Acad. Méd. Paris* **9**, 1235–1236 (1880).

Laveran, A., *Traite des fievres palustres.* Paris: Octave Doin, 1884.

Laveran, A. and Lucet, G., Deux hématozoaires de la perdrix et du dindon, *C.R. Acad. Sci. Paris* **141**, 673–676 (1905).

Lawrence, J. J. and Bearup, A. J., A new host record for *Plasmodium relictum*: the silver gull (*Larus novae-hollandiae* Stephens), *Indian J Malariol.* **15**, 11–19 (1961).

Levine, N. D., Geographic host distribution of blood parasites in columborid birds, *Trans. III. St. Acad. Sci.* **55**, 92–111 (1962).

Lucena, D. T., Malária aviária, *Journal do Commercio*, Recife, Brazil. 1939, 296 pp.

MacCallum, W. G., On the haematozoan infections of birds, *Johns Hopkins Hosp. Bull.* **80**, 235–236 (1897).

Manson, P., The rôle of the mosquito in the evolution of the malarial parasite. The recent researches of Surgeon-Major Ronald Ross, I.M.S., *The Lancet*, August 20, 1898 Vol. II, pp. 488–489.

Manson-Bahr, P. H. and Alcock, A., *The Life and Work of Sir Patrick Manson*. London: Cassell & Co. Ltd, 1927.

Manuel, M. F. and Dulay, A. C., Experimental infection of turkeys with *Plasmodium juxtanucleare*, *Philipp. J. Vet. Med.* **8**, 47–53 (1970).

Manuel, M. F., Tongson, M. S. and Balediata, E. B., Further studies on *Plasmodium juxtanucleare* Versiani and Gomes 1941 in domestic chickens in the Philippines, *Philipp. J. Vet. Med.* **7**, 1–16 (1969).

Manwell, R. D., How many species of avian malaria parasite are there?, *J. Parasitol.* **20**, 334 (1934).

Manwell, R. D., *Plasmodium vaughani* (Novy and MacNeal), *Am. J. Hyg.* **21**, 180–187 (1935a).

Manwell, R. D., How many species of avian malaria parasite are there?, *Amer. J. Trop. Med.* **15**, 265–283 (1935b).

Manwell, R. D., *Plasmodium oti* and *P. hexamerium, J. Parasitol.* **35**, 561–565 (1949).

Manwell, R. D., The blood protozoa of seventeen species of sparrows and other Fringillidae, *J. Protozool.* **2**, 85–86 (1955).

Manwell, R. D., *Plasmodium japonicum, P. juxtanucleare* and *P. nucleophilum* in the Far East, *J. Protozool.* **13**, 8–11 (1966).

Manwell, R. D., *Plasmodium octamerium* n.sp., an avian malaria parasite from the pintail whydah bird *Vidua macroura, J. Protozool.* **15**, 680–685 (1968).

Manwell, R. D., Allen, C. S. and Kuntz, R. E., Blood parasites of Taiwan birds, *J. Protozool.* **23**, 571–576 (1976).

Manwell, R. D. and Kuntz, R. E., *Plasmodium hegneri* n.sp. from the European teal *Anas c. crecca* in Taiwan, *J. Protozool.* **13**, 437–440 (1966).

Manwell, R. D. and Rossi, G. S., Blood protozoa of imported birds, *J. Protozool.* **22**, 124–127 (1975).

Manwell, R. D. and Voter, M. A., Periodicity in the asexual cycle of *Plasmodium nucleophilum* with additional notes on this species, *Am. J. Trop. Med.* **19**, 531–544 (1939).

Marchiafava, E. and Celli, A., Weitere Untersuchungen über die Malariainfektion, *Fortschr. Med.* **3**, 787–792 (1885).

McClure, H. E., *Migration and Survival of the Birds of Asia.* United States Army Medical Component, South-East Asia Treaty Organization (SEATO) Medical Project, Bangkok, Thailand, 1974.

McClure, H. E., Poonswad, P., Greiner, E. C., and Laird, M., *Haematozoa in the Birds of Eastern and Southern Asia.* Memorial University of Newfoundland, St John's, Newfoundland, Canada. 1978, 296 pp.

Mégroz, R. L., *Ronald Ross: Discoverer and Creator*. London: Allen & Unwin, 1931.

Meyer, C. L. and Bennett, G. F., Observations on the sporogony of *Plasmodium circumflexum* Kikuth and *Plasmodium polare* Manwell in New Brunswick, *Can. J. Zool.* **54**, 133–141 (1976).

Mohammed, A. H. H., *Systematic and Experimental Studies on Protozoal Blood Parasites of Egyptian Birds*, Vol. I. Cairo: Cairo University Press, 1958.

Mohan, R. N. and Manwell, R. D., *Plasmodium juxtanucleare* in African partridges (*Francolinus* sp.), *J. Parasitol.* **55**, 543 (1969).

Nandi, N. C., Blood parasites of Indian avifauna. Ph.D. Thesis, University of Calcutta, 1978.

Neill, W. T., *The Geography of Life*. New York–London: Columbia University Press, 1969.

Ogaki, M., Bird malaria parasites found in the Malay Peninsula, *Am. J. Trop. Med.* **29**, 459–462 (1949).

Ogawa, M., Notizen über die blutparasitischen Protozoen bei japanischen Vogeln, *Arch. f. Protistenk.* **24**, 119–125 (1912).

Opie, E., On the hematozoa of birds, *J. Exp. Med.* **3**, 79–101 (1898).

Parkes, K. C., The red junglefowl of the Philippines — native or introduced?, *Auk* **79**, 479–481 (1962).

Raffaele, G., Sul comportamento degli sporozoiti nel sangue dell' ospite, *Riv. di Malariol.* **13**, 395–403 (1934).

Rahal, E. M., Bishop, M. A. and Bennett, G. F., Avian Haemoproteidae. 25. The haemoproteids of the avian family Pycnonotidae (bulbuls), *Can. J. Zool.* **65**, 322–328 (1986).

Ray, A. P., Menon, M. K., Bhatnagar, V. N., Narayandas, M. G. and Chandrasekhar, G. R., Avian *Plasmodium in* Indian birds (*P. polare*), Part II, *Indian J. Malariol.* **7**, 249–252 (1953).

Ross, R., On some peculiar pigmented cells found in two mosquitoes fed on malarial blood, *Br. Med. J.* **2**, 1786–1788 (1897).

Ross, R., *Report on the Cultivation of* Proteosoma, *Labbé, in Grey Mosquitoes.* Calcutta, Govt. Press, May 21, 1898. *According to Mégroz, 1931, "circulated privately, but not allowed to be issued till Oct. 1898". Reprinted in* Indian Medical Gazette, *November/December, 1898.*

Ross, R., *Mosquito Brigades and How to Organise Them.* London: G. Phillip & Son, 1902.

Ross, R., Ed., *Letters from Rome on Certain Discoveries Connected with Malaria.* London: Harrison & Sons, 1929.

Russell, P. F., Avian malaria studies. IV. *Haemoproteus* and *Plasmodium* in birds of Luzon, Philippine Islands, *Philipp. J. Sci.* **48**, 263–268 (1932a).

Russell, P. F., Avian malaria studies. V. *Plasmodium capistrani* sp. nov., an avian malaria parasite in the Philippines, *Philipp. J. Sci.* **48**, 269–289 (1932b).

Russell, P. F., *Man's Mastery of Malaria*, London: Oxford University Press, 1955.

Sandosham, A. A., Bennett, G. F., Yap, L. F. and Omar, E. I., A *Plasmodium* sp. from a glossy tree-starling (*Aplonis panayensis strigatus*), *Singapore Med. J.* **6**, 8–9 (1965).

Sarkar, A. C. and Ray, H. N., A new malarial parasite, *Plasmodium (Garnhamella) conturnixae* [sic] n.subgen., n.sp. from black breasted quail, *Coturnix coromandelica.* (Aves: Galliformes), in *Proc. 3rd Int. Congr. Protozool.*, Leningrad, 1969, pp. 353–354.

Sarkar, A. C. and Ray, H. N., A malarial parasite (*Plasmodium (Garnhamella) coturnixae*) of the grey quail *Coturnix coromandelica (Gmelin). Aves-Galliformes, Ceylon J. Med. Sci.* **21**, 85–91 (1972).

Scott, H. H., Report on the deaths occurring in the Society's Gardens during the year 1926, *Proc. Zool. Soc. Lond.* 173–198 (1927).

Scott, H. H., Report on the deaths occurring in the Society's Gardens during the year 1927, *Proc. Zool. Soc. Lond.* 81–89 (1928).

Seed, T. M. and Manwell, R. D., Plasmodia of birds, in *Parasitic Protozoa,* Vol. III: *Gregarines, Haemogregarines, Coccidia, Plasmodia, and Haemoproteids.* New York: Academic Press, 1977.

Shortt, H. E., Fairley, N. H., Covell, G., Shute, P. G. and Garnham, P. C. C., The pre-erythrocytic stages of *Plasmodium falciparum, Trans. R. Soc. Trop. Med. Hyg.* **44**, 405–419 (1951).

Shortt, H. E. and Garnham, P. C. C., The pre-erythrocytic development of *Plasmodium cynomogli* and *Plasmodium vivax. Trans. R. Soc. Trop. Med. Hyg.* **41**, 785–795 (1948).

Shortt, H. E., Menon, K. P. and Iyer, P. B. S., The natural host of *Plasmodium gallinaceum* (Brumpt, 1935), *J. Malar. Inst. India* **4**, 175–178 (1941).

Sibley, C. G., Ahlquist, J. E. and Monroe, B. L., Jr, A classification of the living birds of the world based on DNA-DNA hybridization studies, *Auk* **105**, 409–423 (1988).

Sibley, C. G. and Monroe, B. L., Jr, *Distribution and Taxonomy of Birds of the World.* New Haven–London: Yale University Press, 1990.

Stephens, J. W. W., A new malaria parasite of man, *Ann. trop. Med. Parasit.* **16**, 383–388 (1922).

Subkhonov, M., Malyar iinye parazity ptits Tadzhikistana [Malaria parasites on the birds of Tadzhikistan], in *Voprosy Zoologii Tadzhikistana*, ed. M. N. Narzikulov and I. A. Abdusalyamov, *Trudy Inst. zool. i parazitol. AN Tadzh. SSR* Donish, Dushanbe, 1972a, pp. 279–286.

Subkhonov, M., Zarazhennost' ptits Tadzhikistana kroveparazitami v zavisimosti ot vremeni goda [Blood parasite infections of birds of Tadzhikistan depending on the time of year], in *Voprosy Zoologii Tadzhikistana*, ed. M. N. Narzikulov and I. A. Abdusalyamov). *Trudy Inst. zool. i parazitol. AN Tadzh. SSR* Donish, Dushanbe, 1972b, pp. 287–293.

Taliaferro, L. G., Infection and resistance in bird malaria with special reference to periodicity and rate of reproduction of the parasites, *Am. J. Hyg.* 5, 742–789 (1925).
Uegaki, J., Untersuchungen über die Blutprotozoen von Vogeln der Sudsee, *Arch. Protistenk* **72**, 74–90 (1930).
van Riper, C., III, Atkinson, C. T. and Seed, T. M., Plasmodia of birds, in *Parasitic Protozoa*, Vol. 7, ed. Kreier, J.P., New York and London: Academic Press, 1994, pp. 73–138.
van Riper, C., III, van Riper, S. G., Goff, M. L. and Laird, M., The epizootiology and ecological significance of malaria in Hawaiian birds, *Ecol. Mgr.* **56**, 327–344 (1986).
Warner, R. E., The role of introduced diseases in the extinction of the endemic Hawaiian avifauna, *Condor* **70**, 101–120 (1968).
Welch, W. H., Malaria: definitions, synonyms, history and parasitology, in Loomis and Thompson's *Syst. Pract. Med.* **I**, 17 (1897).
Whistler, H. *Popular Handbook of Indian Birds*, 4th ed. London: Gurney & Jackson, 1949.
Williams, N. A., Bennett, G. F. and Troncy, P. M., Avian haematozoa of some birds from Tchad, *J. Wildl. Dis.* **13**, 59–61 (1977).
Wolfson, F., Synchronicity, periodicity, and the length of the asexual cycle of *Plasmodium rouxi* in the canary, *Am. J. Hyg.* **23**, 340–348 (1936a).
Wolfson, F., *Plasmodium oti* n.sp., a plasmodium from the eastern screech-owl (*Otus asio naevius*) infective to canaries, *Am. J. Hyg.* **24**, 94–101 (1936b).
Wolfson, F., A strain of *Plasmodium praecox (relictum)* with highly synchronous matinal sporulation, *Am. J. Hyg.* **25**, 177–186 (1937).
Yakunin, M. P., Paraziticheskie prosteishie krovi dikikh ptits Kazakhstana [Parasitic protozoa in the blood of wild birds from Kazakhstan], *Materialy II Vsesoyuzs" ezda protozoologov Naukova Dumka Kiev* **1**, 166–167 (1976).
Yakunin, M. P. and Zhazyltaev, T. A., Parazitofauna krovi dikikh i domashnikh ptits Kazakhstane [The blood parasite fauna of wild and domestic birds from Kazakhstan], *Tr. Inst. zool. Akad. nauk Kaz. SSR* **37**, 124–148 (1977).
Zeiniev, N. R., Kroveparazity ptits severo-vostochnogo Azerbaidzhana [Blood parasites of birds from north-eastern Azerbaidzhan], *Avtoreferat dissertatsii. Inst. zool. AN Azerb. SSR, Baku.* 1–20 (1975a).
Zeiniev, N. R., Paraziticheskie prosteishie krovi ptits severo-vostochnogo Azerbaidzhana [Parasitic protozoa in the blood of birds from north-eastern Azerbaidzhan], *Izv. Akad. nauk Az. SSR, Ser. Biol. Nauk* **4**, 86–89 (1975b).
Zeuner, F. E., *A History of Domesticated Animals*. London: Hutchinson, 1963.